Private Medical Insurance in the United Kingdom

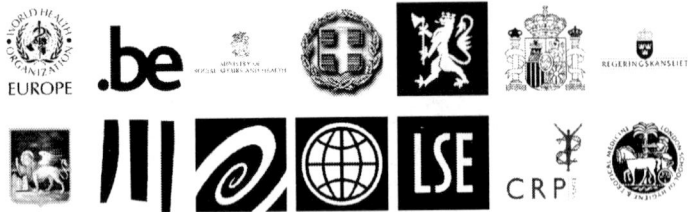

The *European Observatory on Health Systems and Policies* supports and promotes evidence-based health policy-making through comprehensive and rigorous analysis of health care systems in Europe. It brings together a wide range of policy-makers, academics and practitioners to analyse trends in health care reform, drawing on experience from across Europe to illuminate policy issues.

The European Observatory on Health Systems and Policies is a partnership between the World Health Organization Regional Office for Europe, the Governments of Belgium, Finland, Greece, Norway, Spain and Sweden, the Veneto Region of Italy, the European Investment Bank, the Open Society Institute, the World Bank, CRP-Santé Luxembourg, the London School of Economics and Political Science, and the London School of Hygiene and Tropical Medicine.

Private Medical Insurance in the United Kingdom

Thomas Foubister
Research Officer, LSE Health and Social Care, London School of Economics and Political Science

Sarah Thomson
Research Officer, LSE Health and Social Care, London School of Economics and Political Science, and Research Associate at the European Observatory on Health Systems and Policies

Elias Mossialos
Brian Abel-Smith Professor of Health Policy, London School of Economics and Political Science, and Research Director at the European Observatory on Health Systems and Policies

Alistair McGuire
Professor of Health Economics, London School of Economics and Political Science

European
Observatory
on Health Systems and Policies

Keywords:
INSURANCE, HEALTH
FINANCING, HEALTH
DELIVERY OF HEALTH CARE
UNITED KINGDOM

ISBN 92 890 2288 4

Printed in Great Britain by The Cromwell Press, Trowbridge, Wilts.

Contents

Preface

This study provides a descriptive overview of the market for supplementary voluntary health insurance (VHI), or private medical insurance (PMI), in the United Kingdom. The structure of the study reflects the three principal dimensions of the market: the product (Chapter 2), demand (Chapter 3) and supply (Chapter 4). An appendix discusses the market for health cash plans, an alternative type of private medical expenses cover with a relatively broad take-up. The Introduction provides the background necessary for understanding the nature and role of the market for PMI.

Despite regularly being presented as the archetypal system of supplementary VHI, little has been written about the market for PMI. Virtually all academic studies of PMI have been survey-based studies of demand, while the market for PMI has been only a marginal consideration in studies of the United Kingdom health-care system. What substantive information is available is confined largely to industry reports (which are not readily available in libraries) and to the specialized financial media.

Our aim in this study is to help to rectify this situation – something we believe has acquired a certain urgency given the strong interest in supplementary VHI that has developed in recent years (in several countries of central and eastern Europe, in particular) and the part that the United Kingdom example has played in this (to take only the most recent instance, the example of the United Kingdom market for PMI was drawn on by the Supreme Court of Canada in its June 2005 ruling on the illegality of Quebec's prohibition of private health insurance for physician and hospital services).

This study is largely descriptive and is not intended to analyse issues of equity and efficiency within the market for PMI, or to look in detail at the equity and efficiency implications of operating a market in VHI alongside the public health care system. Nevertheless, in the concluding section we briefly highlight some key points that emerge from the study and that might be of interest to decision-makers interested in developing or extending a supplementary VHI market. We also provide a short glossary of the key terms used.

Although this overview of the market attempts to be comprehensive, there are several important areas that we have been unable to address in detail. These include the "self-pay" market for private medical services (which may affect demand for PMI) and the private provider market (which does affect how the PMI industry operates). To have looked at these issues in depth would have opened our topic up to encompass the private health care market as a whole, and this was not a practical option. The other area of significance that we would have liked to have addressed is the issue of premium inflation. There is a consensus that premiums have been rising at rates significantly higher than general inflation for many years, and that this is dampening demand. The factors that underpin premium inflation are well known: rising claims frequency on the back of new technologies, the need to maintain margins at adequate levels, and so on. However, there are no publicly available data on premium inflation in the United Kingdom market – the industry premium income figures that are available are aggregated for the market as a whole and for all products, and capture neither instances of product up- or downgrading, nor whether cover is extended to subscriber dependants or not. Thus, although these figures can tell us how much more subscribers in the aggregate are willing to spend on insurance on a year-to-year basis, they do not tell us anything about how much a given amount of insurance has changed in price. Further research in this area requires the cooperation of insurers.

Thomas Foubister
Sarah Thomson
Elias Mossialos
Alistair McGuire

Acknowledgements

This study is based on information available in the public domain. Searches included the following resources: the World Wide Web; academic databases including PubMed, IBSS and EconLit; the mainstream press and the financial press; insurer web sites and product-related documentation; company annual reports held at Companies House; human resources reports; the Consumer Association and Chartered Insurance Institute materials pertaining to PMI; and data from the Organisation for Economic Co-operation and Development (OECD), the Department of Health, the Office for National Statistics, and Centers for Medicare and Medicaid Services (United States).

Our primary source of information on the PMI industry (the composition of the industry, recent industry developments, market performance, and trends in subscriber numbers) has been the report produced annually by the industry analyst Laing & Buisson. Other industry reports were consulted, but it was decided that they would remain supplementary to our main source. We are grateful to Laing & Buisson for granting us permission to reproduce their data.

One of the main obstacles to research into PMI is the absence of disaggregated data. We attempted, via a detailed questionnaire, to obtain data necessary to provide a substantive description of market activity, but the PMI Committee of the Association of British Insurers (on which all the major private medical insurers sit) told us that companies were unable to respond to the questionnaire because of a lack of resources. We have therefore had to rely largely on data aggregated for the market as a whole.

We are grateful to the representatives of AXA PPP, BUPA, Norwich Union Healthcare and Standard Life Healthcare, who agreed to speak to us. Our intention in speaking to insurers was solely to seek verification for our own interpretation of market developments and to gain a general sense of the industry's impression of the recent and possible future evolution of the market. Accordingly, we have chosen not to draw on anything said during these conversations here. We would also like to thank the Association of British Insurers for facilitating our contact with the industry, and for lending us its support in our efforts to gather information.

The research on which this study is based was funded by the United Kingdom Department of Health (grant reference number 0300090), to whom we are grateful. We would also like to thank members of the Department of Health and Professor Alan Maynard for their feedback. Needless to say, this study represents the authors' interpretation of the market alone, and the authors are fully responsible for any errors.

Executive Summary

The principal type of voluntary health insurance (VHI) operating in the United Kingdom is supplementary VHI, or private medical insurance (PMI). PMI provides insured access to privately delivered care that duplicates many of the services provided by the National Health Service (NHS) (to which PMI subscribers retain full access). The key attractions of PMI vis-à-vis the NHS are faster access to treatment, a more comfortable care environment, and a wider choice of specialists, treatment facilities and timing of treatment. Although the public and private sectors are relatively well integrated on the delivery side of the health care system, PMI and public funding operate as distinct, unrelated streams of health-care finance.

The product

PMI provides cover for the costs of treatment for acute conditions and for the costs of related services such as accommodation, nursing and – where relevant – outpatient services. PMI products may offer cover beyond these core benefits, however, with a broader scope being reflected in a higher price.

There are two PMI submarkets: the individual market and the corporate market. In the corporate market, PMI is employer-purchased, and is provided to employees as a work-related benefit. In about 12.5% of company schemes, the employer requires employees to make a contribution to the premium (AON Consulting, 2004).

In the individual market and part of the corporate market (usually companies of fewer than 50 employees), PMI is underwritten; in the larger part of the corporate market, it is not. Underwriting is the process by which the insurer decides the risk that it is willing to assume. Insurers usually exclude from cover all pre-existing conditions (we define pre-existing conditions as conditions present at application, but insurers may extend its meaning to include past conditions, or those present during a specified number of years prior to application). These are excluded because the need for treatment is approaching certainty, and insurance only functions when there is uncertainty around the likelihood of treatment being required.

After the exclusion of pre-existing conditions, insurers use two principal forms of underwriting: full medical underwriting and moratorium underwriting. Full medical underwriting requires the applicant to provide details of his/her medical history; on the basis of this information, the insurers will determine what is to be excluded – e.g. previous conditions that might re-emerge, or conditions that might emerge in future as a result of previous conditions or of pre-existing conditions. Again, the reason for these exclusions is the difficulty faced by insurers in pricing high-risk events. However, it also avoids attracting subscribers who are already ill or who have been ill in the past (it being against the interest of insurers to attract subscribers with a high probability of having to make a claim, because of the more-or-less inevitable imprecision involved in pricing by risk).

With moratorium underwriting, the process described above is shifted to the point of claim. Here, conditions suffered in the five years prior to insurance purchase are automatically excluded from cover for two years, as are any directly related conditions. If the subscriber is symptom-free and has not sought advice or treatment for the condition or related conditions during the moratorium period, cover commences. Presentation of symptoms or receipt of advice or treatment during the moratorium period means that the two years must begin anew.

Insurers price the premium to reflect the risk presented by the subscriber. The most important risk category is age. The risk presented (the likelihood of having to make a claim) increases with age, and therefore older subscribers are charged a higher premium than younger ones. Other categories, such as gender, occupational status and smoking status, may be used. Insurers are beginning to incorporate further risk factors, such as height and weight characteristics. In the main part of the corporate market, there is generally no underwriting, and the premium is priced to reflect the company's claims experience in the previous year.

There are four basic dimensions of price. The first is the scope of cover chosen, the second is the risk profile of the applicant (or claims experience in the corporate market), the third comprises the product options attached to the basic product (principally constraints on how the product can be used, and cost sharing), and the fourth is the loading charge (the costs accrued by the insurer in fulfilling its function as insurer, plus profit).

There are three product types, which differ by the degree to which the scope of cover they offer extends beyond the basic acute care benefits common to all PMI products. These are comprehensive, standard and budget policies. Comprehensive policies are the most expensive, and include a relatively wide range of benefits. Budget policies are the cheapest, offering a narrower range of benefits and may also involve some automatic constraints on usage.

There are some items that may not be covered under any policy. These include pre-existing medical conditions, but also conditions and services that place insurers at high risk of moral hazard and those that are especially resource-intensive. Under insurance, claims probabilities have to be independent of one another – a provider of PMI will also, therefore, withdraw cover when claims are interdependent, that is, where a large proportion of subscribers may have to claim simultaneously as a result of the same single causal factor (war or conditions related to a mass accident, for example). This is to protect the insurer from collapse.

Once an individual has chosen the level of cover required, he/she can choose options that will affect the price of the product. The most important of these are the choice to extend cover to dependants (this raises the price), constraints on the choice of hospital, and cost sharing (these lower the price, as they represent a cost saving – for the insurer – that can be passed on to the subscriber). In the corporate market, some 63% of schemes restrict access to hospitals according to whether or not they are on a list of those with which the insurer has negotiated a discount (AON Health Solutions, 2002), and some 43.5% of employers operate an excess (AON Consulting, 2004) – the usual level being between £51 and £100 per claim (AON Health Solutions, 2002).

There may be problems of clarity regarding precisely what is or is not covered by a policy, whether this is prior to the point of purchase, when products are being compared, or at the point of claim. The choice of product (comprehensive, standard or budget) and product options, general exclusions, and underwriting all affect what will be covered. On top of this integral complexity, insurers differ in their use of terminology, or may be unclear about what they mean by certain specific key terms such as "acute condition", "pre-existing condition", "chronic condition", and so on.

Problems centring around clarity, competition through product differentiation, and the proliferation of products and product options available have led to concerns regarding the possibility of consumer detriment. In the 1990s, the Office of Fair Trading (OFT) conducted two investigations into the market, and criticized the industry for the following: lack of terminological clarity and difficulty of product comparability; the use of moratorium underwriting (which risks confusing the consumer and, at worst, giving the consumer an incentive to forgo seeking medical advice); and the absence of provision of information about premium inflation.

In 2000, self-regulation was established in the form of the General Insurance Standards Council (GISC). This organization implemented a Practice Requirement for PMI in 2004, which sought to address some of these concerns and to help reduce consumer detriment by improving the sales process and the presentation of product information. The GISC was disbanded in January 2005, as regulation of sales was assumed by the Financial Services Authority (FSA) – the first time that insurance sales had been subject to external, statutory regulation.

Regulation under the FSA focuses on ensuring that the sales process is transparent and that the information needed for the consumer to assess the product is presented clearly and consistently across insurers and across products. Given its focus on the sales process alone, regulation by the FSA may be limited in terms of eliminating consumer detriment resulting from the nature of competition within this market. But, because of the nature of the administrative burden it places on sales, this regulation may have some indirect material impact on product design that would be beneficial to the consumer.

In the past, product development has been focused on providing product options that allow the consumer to lower the price of his/her cover. Recent developments in the corporate market have seen the focus placed on health promotion and on illness prevention. Developments in the individual market, meanwhile, have seen PMI being combined with other forms of health care payment and with other forms of insurance – a move that may signal more complexity in individual-market product design.

Demand for private medical insurance

Table 1 presents data, for 1997–2003, on the number of subscribers to PMI in the individual market, the corporate market and the total market, and the number of people covered as a percentage of the United Kingdom population for the total market.

Since the early 1990s, about 11.5% of the United Kingdom population (including dependants of subscribers) has had some form of PMI cover. Over this period, subscriber numbers in the individual market have been

Table 1 *Subscriber numbers and people covered, as a percentage of the United Kingdom population, 1997–2003* (Source: *Laing & Buisson, 2004*)

| | Subscriber Numbers (millions) | | | |
Year	*Individual market*	*Corporate market*	*Total market*	*People covered (% of UK population)*
1997	1.378	2.108	3.486	11.6
1998	1.335	2.250	3.585	11.7
1999	1.285	2.275	3.560	11.2
2000	1.242	2.437	3.679	11.7
2001	1.216	2.506	3.722	11.3
2002	1.193	2.515	3.709	11.4
2003	1.157	2.514	3.671	11.2

declining steadily, with subscriber numbers in the corporate market rising steadily. However, in 2003, numbers in the corporate market contracted for the first time since 1994, and the overall market saw a contraction in the subscriber base of 1.02%.

Subscribers to PMI tend to share certain characteristics across the following parameters: age (demand for PMI is highest among those aged 55–64); income (higher-income individuals are more likely to have PMI); educational level (those with post-secondary school education are more likely to have PMI); employment status (those in higher-level occupations or roles are more likely to have PMI); area of residence (those in the south-east, the east and London are more likely to have PMI); and political attitude (Conservative voters are more likely to have PMI).

The two most important supply-side factors affecting demand for PMI are perceptions of NHS quality and the price of PMI. Studies looking at the relationship between waiting lists/times and demand for PMI find that there is some connection between the two, although it may be that perceptions of waiting lists are more important than the reality of waiting lists or the experience of having had to wait. Regarding price, continuous above-inflation price rises appear to have placed downward pressure on demand for PMI over time, while the removal of tax subsidies for the over-60s in the individual market appears to have had only a minor effect in terms of reducing demand, suggesting that in this market the use of tax subsidies is ineffective and an inefficient use of resources.

The industry

There are currently 27 insurers operating in the United Kingdom market for

PMI, as well as several PMI carriers without an underwriting capacity of their own (Laing & Buisson, 2004). The share of the market between provident companies and commercial companies is roughly 50:50 (although the distinction appears to be a formal one only, as market behaviour appears to be similar regardless of legal status).

The most important industry development during the 1990s was the market entry of commercial companies. The most important recent development has been the entry of insurers on an underwriting-only basis, and the entry of PMI carriers without an underwriting capacity of their own. Since the early 1990s, the market has been characterized by a relatively high level of entry and exit, suggesting that entry costs are moderate (particularly in the individual market), and also that it has proved difficult for new entrants to make inroads into the market shares held by the established providers.

A recent development in the corporate market has been the rapid growth of non-insured medical expenses schemes (NIMES – a form of company "self-insurance"). Here, enrolee numbers have grown from 53 000 in 1992 to 472 000 in 2003 (Laing & Buisson, 2004), representing a threat to the potential for growth in the corporate market for PMI. However, insurers have been taking advantage of this growth area by offering services as administrators of NIMES.

Intermediaries operate primarily in the corporate market: about 74% of corporate market sales were intermediated in 2003 (Laing & Buisson, 2004). Intermediaries operating in the individual market do so largely on an accommodation basis (dealing with existing customers rather than new ones). Of all PMI sales in 2003, some 53% were intermediated, and, of these, some 90% were corporate market sales (Laing & Buisson, 2004).

In 2003, about 85% of individual market PMI sales were made direct to the consumer (Laing & Buisson, 2004), on the back of advertising and through insurer sales staff. Expenditure on advertising varies among insurers, with the British United Provident Association (BUPA) leading in 2002 with an expenditure of £11.831 million (Datamonitor, 2003).

The top four market players – BUPA, AXA PPP, Norwich Union Healthcare and Standard Life Healthcare – have dominated the market continuously, with 78% of the market between them in 2003 (Laing & Buisson, 2004). Following these four are several insurers with an established historical presence and smaller, but stable, market shares. BUPA is the clear leader in terms of market share. Although BUPA's share of the market dipped after 1992, it began to rise again in the second half of the 1990s to stand at 40% of the market in 2003. AXA PPP follows, having a 22.5% market share (Laing & Buisson, 2004).

In terms of relationships with providers of medical care, insurer market power appears to matter. Insurers negotiate discounts with providers, which they can then pass on to their customers in the form of reduced premiums or as hospital network options. Insurers reimburse provider facilities directly; however, the specialist fee is usually charged to the subscriber, who will then be reimbursed by the insurer. Insurers have fee schedules and will usually not reimburse specialist fees that are in excess of these schedules, it being up to the subscriber to make up any shortfall.

Table 2 provides data on premium income and claims expenditure aggregated for the whole market for 1997–2003, and also shows rates of growth (adjusted for the retail price index (RPI)).

Despite a largely static subscriber base, premium income has exceeded growth in claims expenditure in all but three two-year clusters in the last 15 years. Given the static subscriber base, growth in premium income has been driven by rises in the price of premiums rather than by attracting new customers into the market.

Growth in claims expenditure has been moderate since 1992, with the exception of the 6% growth rate in 1999. In 2003, growth was at its lowest in recent history, at 0.8%. This may mean that insurer efforts to contain growth (through provider negotiation, through the sale of downgraded products, and through some managed-care or utilization-review techniques – plus the recent focus, in the corporate market, on health promotion and detecting ill health early) are beginning to pay off.

Since the late 1970s, gross margins (the excess of premium income over claims expenditure) were at their highest in 2003, at some 23.6% (aggregated for the industry as a whole). Gross margins are significantly higher in the individual market than in the corporate market, largely because of the much higher level of competition in the corporate market and the ability of insurers to pass on premium increases in the individual market without adverse levels of subscriber loss (demand for PMI being particularly price-inelastic in the individual market). Table 3 shows gross margins, broken down by submarket, for 1997–2003.

Gross margins include administrative costs and profit. Profit also derives from the investment of premium income in the stock market, and, when the market is strong, returns on this investment can allow insurers to make a profit even when losing money on their insurance business. Profit levels measured as a percentage of premium income vary between insurers, and also vary within the same insurer on a year-to-year basis. Administrative costs as a percentage of premium income vary significantly from insurer to insurer, but appear to be relatively stable on a year-to-year basis.

Table 2 *Premium income and claims expenditure, 1997–2003 (Source: Laing & Buisson, 2004)*

Year	Premium income (£ millions)	Premium-income growth (real) (%)	Claims expenditure (£ millions)	Claims-expenditure growth (real) (%)
1997	1 999	3.5	1 586	2.4
1998	2 071	0.2	1 703	3.9
1999	2 224	5.7	1 834	6.0
2000	2 456	7.3	1 943	2.9
2001	2 661	6.4	2 069	4.6
2002	2 862	5.8	2 205[a]	4.4
2003	2 978	1.1	N/A	0.8

N/A, not applicable.
[a] Estimated value.

Table 3 *Industry gross margins, 1997–2003 (Source: authors' calculations based on figures provided in Laing & Buisson, 2004)*

	Gross Margins (%)	
Year	Individual market	Corporate market
1997	26.1	14.7
1998	21.7	13.8
1999	21.1	13.9
2000	26.7	14.9
2001	24.9	19.8
2002	25.7	20.4
2003	N/A	N/A

N/A, not applicable.

The market for health cash plans

Health cash plans provide reimbursement for out-of-pocket expenditure on health care and related items. The benefits paid are fixed monetary amounts, and are very small compared with the reimbursement provided by PMI (there may be an annual maximum benefit of, for example, £100 for a given service). In 2003, there were some 2.892 million subscribers to health cash plans, with some 4.796 million people being covered. This represented a decline, however, on 2002, when there were 2.976 million subscribers and 5.097 million people covered (Laing & Buisson, 2004). Nevertheless, as subscriber numbers declined in 2003, premium income grew at the high rate of 7.5% (Laing & Buisson, 2004). This shows that, at these low price levels (health cash plans may cost as little as £1 per week), the market readily absorbs price increases.

There are 35 providers of health cash plans, some eight of whom also provide PMI. Twenty-three of these providers are provident associations (Laing &

Buisson, 2004). In 2003, gross margins (aggregated for the industry) were 29.1%, an increase of 2.3 percentage points on 2002. The bulk of this increase in gross margins appears to have gone to the largest provider of health cash plans, HSA (Laing & Buisson, 2004).

Chapter 1

Introduction

Understanding voluntary health insurance: a functional classification

The need for a shared terminology

Most countries operate mixed systems of health care financing, combining out-of-pocket spending, private health insurance, and public funding (tax financing or social health insurance) (Mossialos & Dixon, 2002). Debate around the financing of health care usually centres on two related issues: the weight that should be accorded each component of the mix, and the way in which these components are best integrated.

In recent years, private health insurance has been gaining ground as a policy option in rich and poor countries alike. Supporters of the trend hold that for rich countries, expanding private health insurance will help governments to contain growth in public spending on health care, while for poor countries it presents the only realistic hope of achieving broad population access to health care on an insured basis.

For critics, the trend goes against the grain of a valued historical trajectory whereby public financing of health care emerged in response to access-related problems arising from the normal operation of private markets in health insurance, namely affordability barriers for the poor – just as, formerly, health insurance had emerged in response to similar problems arising from the operation of health care markets based on out-of-pocket spending, namely, affordability barriers for the ill.

It is not our aim to explore these arguments here, but we would note that the progress of the debate around the merits of enhancing the role of private health insurance has, in our view, been hampered by the absence of a simple shared terminology (something that has also increased the risk of inappropriate policy choices being made). In this section, we present a classification of the various forms of VHI – private health insurance the purchase of which is voluntary rather than mandated – which we hope will serve as a reference point for those debating the operation, introduction or extension of markets in VHI. Our immediate aim, however, is to introduce the principal form of VHI in operation in the United Kingdom.

The United Kingdom combines public sector and private sector involvement on both the financing and delivery sides of health care, and the relationships between the different components of this mix are complex. We then outline the United Kingdom's mixed economy of health provision, with the aim of showing how the VHI market fits into the health care system as a whole.

Drivers of market development

There are three types of VHI (Mossialos & Thomson, 2004): complementary VHI, substitutive VHI, and supplementary VHI. The type of VHI that develops in a country will be determined by the nature of the publicly financed component of that country's health care system (referred to here as "the public system").

There are four aspects of the public system that are of special importance in establishing the range of opportunities available to insurers for the development of a market in VHI. We term these the core drivers of VHI market development. These are outlined below.

- *Scope of coverage* (benefits covered by the public system). What is included and what is not included in the benefits package, or, where there is no defined benefits package, realistically, what can be expected to be covered?

- *Depth of coverage* (the proportion of benefit cost met by the public system). Are benefits fully covered, or does the user of health care have to make a financial contribution at the point of use?

- *System inclusiveness* (the proportion of the population to which coverage is extended). Is coverage universal, or are groups excluded from, or allowed to opt out of, being eligible to receive and – usually – having to pay for health care within the public system?

- *Consumer satisfaction* (perceptions about quality of care). Is there dissatisfaction with the public system, in conjunction with willingness to pay for privately financed health care over and above the mandatory contribution made to the public system?

Collectively, these drivers can be gathered under the heading "gaps in coverage" (that is, gaps in terms of services, costs, people and expectations). The three types of VHI correspond to the four drivers of market development: complementary VHI to the first two, substitutive VHI to the third, and supplementary VHI to the fourth. These are described in turn below.

The three types of voluntary health insurance

Complementary voluntary health insurance

Complementary VHI arises to address deficiencies in scope and depth of coverage within the public system. Regarding scope of coverage, public systems are increasingly choosing to exclude services that might, under more favourable resource conditions, have reasonably been included in the public benefits package (a typical example being dental care). Where this is taking place, markets in complementary VHI may emerge to facilitate access to such care on an insured basis. This type of complementary VHI is found, for example, covering dental care in the Netherlands and Spain (Mossialos & Thomson, 2004).

Regarding depth of coverage, public systems might require patients to pay a user charge when accessing care (an example might be a flat fee payable when visiting a general practitioner (GP) or specialist). Again, markets in complementary VHI may emerge to enable patients to pay such charges on an insured basis. This type of complementary VHI is found, for example, in France (Mossialos & Thomson, 2004).

In summary, when public coverage is incomplete in terms of scope or depth of coverage, a market for VHI that complements (in the sense of completes) the public system may develop.

Substitutive voluntary health insurance

Substitutive VHI addresses deficiencies in system inclusiveness. In some countries, certain population groups (for instance, individuals with an annual income above a threshold, or those below a specified age) may be excluded from, or allowed to opt out of, the public system. Markets in substitutive VHI develop to make it possible for these groups to access health care on an insured basis. Substitutive VHI is thus so-called because it substitutes for (i.e. takes the place of) the public system, and is found in, for example, Germany, the Netherlands (Mossialos & Thomson, 2004) and the United States.

Markets in substitutive VHI will tend to offer packages that provide a level of cover broadly comparable to that offered by the parallel public system. However, they may also offer a range of alternative packages, some of which will cover a more limited range of services (those that might be considered "essential", for instance), and some of which will cover a wider range of services. Different packages may also require higher or lower levels of cost sharing. Differences in package design such as these will be reflected in the price of the premium.

Supplementary voluntary health insurance

Supplementary VHI arises to address instances of low levels of consumer satisfaction with the public system, and is designed to provide alternative insured access to health care. Markets in supplementary VHI will arise where low levels of consumer satisfaction are coupled with willingness to pay for privately financed health care, over and above the mandatory contribution made to the public system (to which full right of access is retained). This is the principal form of VHI operating in the United Kingdom.

There are several possible causes of low levels of consumer satisfaction with publicly financed health care. In terms of the development of markets in supplementary VHI, the most important causes are those that relate to what might broadly be described as non-clinical dimensions of quality. These include the presence of waiting times, unhappiness with the care environment (ward accommodation, impersonal service or unattractive surroundings) and restrictions on product availability (for instance, non-coverage of a brand-name drug that the patient would choose over the available generic version under conditions more favourable to the exercise of consumer choice).

Like substitutive VHI, supplementary VHI is offered in various packages, each having a different scope and depth of coverage; these differences are again reflected in the price of the premium. Supplementary VHI usually covers many of the services covered by the public system – this being referred to sometimes as its duplicatory function (Colombo & Tapay, 2004) – while seeking to maintain non-clinical dimensions of quality at a comparatively high level. It may also extend cover to benefits that are excluded from the public system, such as access to alternative therapies (here, supplementary VHI might be thought of as partially serving a "complementary" function). More restrictive packages might be limited to services for which, for example, there are long waits in the public system (these are among the less-expensive products available on the United Kingdom market). Alternatively, they may be limited to providing cover for the so-called "top-up" benefits, such as access to superior accommodation (this type of package has thus far been unable to develop in the United Kingdom owing to restrictions on how private and public flows of funds can be combined, but it does exist elsewhere in Europe).

There are two classes of benefit, however, to which supplementary VHI will not usually extend cover. The first concerns benefits that are particularly resource-intensive, such as accident and emergency services. The second concerns those benefits that insurers perceive to place them at high risk of moral hazard (where being insured alters the behaviour of the individual in such a way as to lead to higher than predicted costs for the insurer). Supplementary VHI will in many cases not, therefore, extend cover to cosmetic surgery, GP visits and pregnancy- and childbirth-related care – all areas over which the individual is held to exert significant control.

Supplementary VHI is not so-called because it is designed to provide cover for items that might be thought of as supplementing those covered by the public system (extra choice, faster access, more comfort). It is so-called, rather, because it is as a system of insurance that it can be thought of as being supplementary to – adding to, but surplus to, while supplanting without constituting a true substitute to – the public system.

Dynamics of voluntary health insurance market development

Insurers that wish to develop a market in VHI will, in the first instance, seek to determine whether any of the four drivers of market development are present. If the public system excludes services valued by consumers concerned about their access to effective health care, or if it imposes a charge for access, there may be potential for the development of a market in complementary VHI. If part of the population is not covered by the public system (or if there is no functional public system), there may be potential for the development of a market in substitutive VHI. Finally, if insurers perceive there to be consumer dissatisfaction with the public system, there may be potential for the development of a market in supplementary VHI.

Where VHI markets are in place, insurers may put pressure on public decision-makers to enhance the core drivers of market development. They may argue, for instance, that where there is an established market in supplementary VHI, beneficiaries should be allowed to opt out of the public system and a substitutive VHI market be encouraged to develop. Or they may argue that the public system should not cover all the benefits that it does cover, and that the market in complementary VHI should be encouraged to expand. Or they may simply set out to stoke consumer dissatisfaction with the public system so as to facilitate the expansion of an existing market in supplementary VHI.

The process also operates in reverse. If a functioning market in complementary VHI exists, public decision-makers concerned with containing costs in the public system may find it easier, politically, to exclude covered items from the public system or to introduce charges for access. Alternatively, if complementary and supplementary VHI markets are already in place, public decision-makers may see potential for the development of a market in substitutive VHI and for allowing groups to opt out of the public system. The same applies where there is only a limited public system. Here, public decision-makers may see the development of a market in substitutive VHI as a means of achieving broad access to health care on an insured basis. Finally, if demand on the public system is seen to be unsustainably high and resistance to the exclusion of benefits strong, public decision-makers might decide to foster the development of a market in supplementary VHI so that pressure on the public system can be eased.

Our point, here, is that the process is a dynamic one. Gaps in public-system coverage will present opportunities for insurers, who may seek to enhance these gaps further through their public relations or lobbying activities. But, at the same time, public decision-makers may seek to take advantage of the existence of, or of the potential for the development of, markets in VHI to widen their own range of opportunities when developing policy on cost containment and other public system-related matters.

This account is not meant to suggest that no other factors come into play. Other important factors, such as the ownership and structure of medical care providers and the way in which governments regulate insurance and health-care markets, will serve to encourage or to constrain the development of a market in VHI. For our present purpose, however, factors such as these have been considered exogenous and have therefore been bracketed.

Note on the classification

An objection may be raised with respect to the above classification – namely, that we have accorded analytical priority to the public system of health care financing. There is, admittedly, an element of arbitrariness to this, but we feel it is justified on two grounds: first, the need to develop a classification that is simple and that serves the intended purpose necessitates some compromise (hence the willingness to refer to VHI as "substitutive" in situations where it is the primary or sole mode of insuring against the costs of health care); and, second, we feel that the historical development of health insurance, which has seen increasing government involvement over time – best understood, perhaps, in terms of "government as the ultimate risk manager" (Moss, 2002) – lends legitimacy to the analytical priority we have accorded the public system. Needless to say, this is not intended to have normative implications.

Voluntary health insurance in the United Kingdom's mixed economy of health

The United Kingdom's mixed economy of health

The principal form of VHI operating in the United Kingdom is supplementary VHI, known there as PMI. This is how it shall be referred to here. PMI is one component of a mixed economy of health which comprises public and private financing and public and private provision. The relationships between these components are complex and are evolving. In this section, we provide a general description of this mixed economy. Because our intention is only to enable the reader to understand how PMI fits into the wider system as a whole, we do not go into the precise details of the operation of the system.

The National Health Service

In the United Kingdom, the bulk of health care financing derives from public funds (see Tables 1.1 and 1.2 below). These funds are allocated by the government to the NHS – and primarily to the major NHS purchasing centres, the Primary Care Trusts (PCTs). PCTs use this funding to purchase services on behalf of the geographically defined populations for which they are responsible. Coverage for health care through the NHS is extended to all those who are "ordinarily resident" in the United Kingdom.

NHS funds flow from PCTs to publicly owned NHS providers and to independent providers. The two principal recipients are the NHS providers and GPs. The former are mainly the NHS Trusts, each of which comprises one or more hospitals and may include other types of facility too. Recently, high-performing NHS Trusts have been granted "Foundation" status, giving them increased independence from the political and administrative centre regarding their financial and management affairs. Nevertheless, they remain publicly owned institutions.

The second major group of recipients of NHS funds are the GPs. Unlike the NHS and Foundation Trusts, GPs are private providers – with one commentator describing them as "small businessmen in the for-profit category" (Saltman, 2003). However, because GPs are required to contract with the NHS alone, they have always been regarded as a constituent part of the NHS. There are other (so-called private) GPs who do not hold contracts to provide NHS-funded care, and these are able to see patients on a private basis. Their number is small, however, and they are paid on an out-of-pocket basis rather than through PMI.

From the early 1980s onwards, the NHS was an occasional purchaser of services from the private sector, when capacity problems in the NHS were deemed sufficiently serious to force it to do so. Such services were purchased largely by NHS providers (this was essentially a form of subcontracting) rather than NHS purchasers. Recently, however, following government policy on waiting times and patient choice, capacity-enhancing arrangements with private sector providers have begun to be formalized (Lewis & Gillam, 2003; Higgins, 2004). Primary Care Trusts are now able to purchase services on a regular or longer-term basis from private sector providers including private hospitals, independent treatment centres, and teams of clinicians from abroad. These different private providers are now, in effect, competing with established NHS providers for the public financing controlled by the Primary Care Trusts. This arrangement, originally intended to constitute a response to short-term capacity problems within the NHS, has become a permanent feature of the health-care system.

In summary, health care administered through the NHS is financed from public funds but is delivered by both publicly owned and privately owned provider institutions. The involvement of the private sector in the delivery of NHS-funded health care is likely to become more significant in coming years.

Private financing of health care

In the last few years of the 1990s, private expenditure accounted for almost 20% of all expenditure on health care. More recently, this figure has declined as a result of the government's decision to inject more resources into the NHS (its intention being to bring United Kingdom health care spending, as a proportion of gross domestic product, up to the European Union average). Nevertheless, the private share of expenditure on health care remains substantial (over 16.5% in 2002) (see Table 1.2).

Public funds flow to both public and private providers. Private funds, in contrast, flow only to private providers (see Figure 1.1). This separation of public and private finance streams is a key feature of the United Kingdom's health care system in its present manifestation. Despite discussion as to whether private funds should be able to flow to NHS providers (for an illustration of the debate, see Richards, Dingwall & Watson, 2001), public providers cannot receive private income. At the same time, private providers delivering services to the NHS cannot combine private revenue and public revenue in the same NHS-contracted service (some private providers are, for the time being, prohibited from receiving any private income at all, thereby avoiding this possibility altogether).

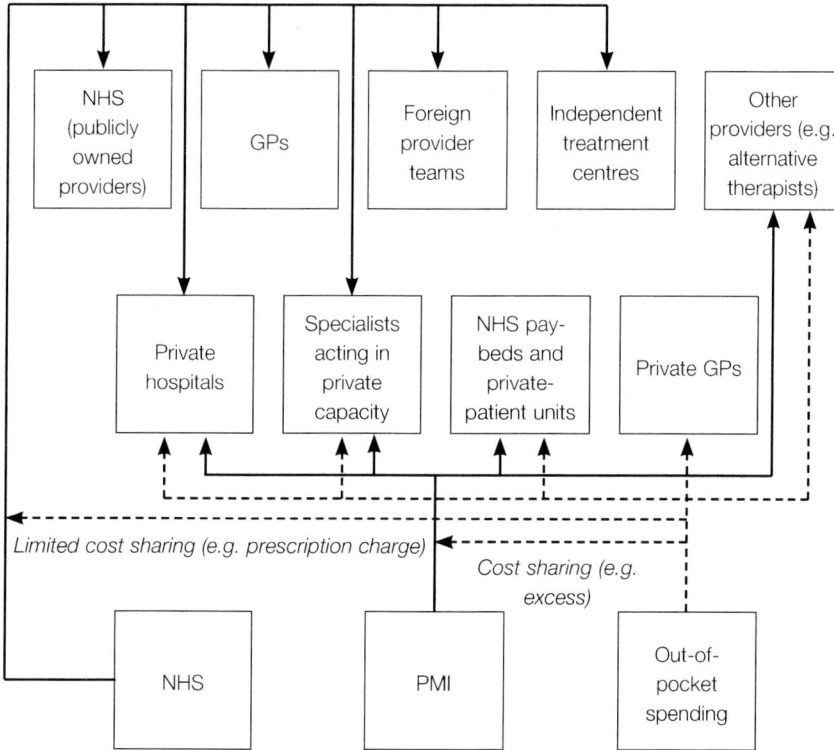

Figure 1.1 *Principal flows of funds in the United Kingdom health-care system*

Note to Figure 1.1: private hospitals and specialists (acting in a private capacity) have been boxed separately, as the initial consultation and the hospital treatment are separated in time and place (moreover, a privately financed consultation may not necessarily lead to a hospital episode). Furthermore, the consultation will often take place in office space that does not belong to a private hospital and for which the specialist will pay rent or a fee.

There are two major exceptions to the "public income only" rule for public providers. The first is the presence of user charges in the NHS. Patients in the United Kingdom are required to pay a flat fee for pharmaceuticals and certain other products or services, a requirement that was put in place very soon after the inception of the NHS in 1948 (Klein, 2001). The system of exemptions is broad, however, with vulnerable members of society not having to pay, so NHS income from this source is correspondingly low.

The second exception to the "public income only" rule is the ability of NHS providers to act in a private capacity. NHS Trusts and Foundation Trusts are allowed to set aside beds, or to put in place dedicated units, for services provided to patients funded on an out-of-pocket or a PMI basis. These "pay-beds" and "private patient units" exist to meet the needs of doctors whose part-time contracts with the NHS allow them to undertake private practice. These practitioners are the people upon whom the operation of the public–private health care mix as a whole depends, as one pool of doctors provides medical services to both sectors. This arrangement also, however, allows the provider to keep these doctors on site, thereby saving on travel time between NHS and private facilities, and to benefit from an additional stream of revenue.

In the 1970s, the Labour Government attempted to abolish pay-beds, in the face of aggressive opposition from the PMI industry. Although the government failed, it did manage to reduce the number of pay-beds significantly. Ironically, however, this (limited) success was to provide the crucial impetus for the expansion of the private hospital industry that the then government found so distasteful (Robb & Brown, 1984). Pay-bed numbers have risen steadily since, and now the NHS actively competes with private hospitals for income from privately financed patients.

Private funding, prohibited from flowing to public providers (unless these providers are acting in a private capacity – in which case the services delivered can be funded through private sources alone), flows principally to private hospitals (independent hospitals and hospitals belonging to private hospital groups) and, to a lesser degree, to NHS pay-beds and private patient units. It is possible that, in future, insurers might also be able to purchase services from the independent treatment centres established to serve the NHS. Insurers are optimistic regarding the potential of these facilities to bring downward pressure to bear on medical inflation in the private provider sector, owing to the economies of scale they operate, and because of the fact that they make less use of higher-cost consultant physicians than do other private providers (Baker, 2004). It is unclear what subscribers to PMI would make of such a development, however, as access to consultant-level physicians and surgeons is an important selling point of PMI.

The contribution of private medical insurance to the health economy

As the figures in Table 1.1 and Table 1.2 show, the financial contribution of PMI to the health economy is small in relation to public spending, and is also small relative to total private spending. Yet, in absolute terms, the contribution of PMI is substantial, standing at £2.86 billion (as measured by premium income) in 2002, and rising some 4% in the space of a year to £2.98 billion in 2003 (Laing & Buisson, 2004). In terms of the share of the population with some form of PMI cover, PMI's contribution to the health economy is more significant still. In 2003, there were 3.76 million subscribers to PMI, with cover being extended to a further 2.875 million individuals (subscribers' dependants) – bringing the total number of individuals with access to private

Table 1.1 *Expenditure on health care by source, 1997–2002 (£ billions)* (Sources: *Lee, Wallis & Heasman, 2004; Office for National Statistics, 2004; Laing & Buisson, 2004*)

Expenditure (£ billions)	1997	1998	1999	2000	2001	2002
Public expenditure	44.568	47.552	52.192	55.996	62.090	67.201
Private expenditure,	10.894	11.626	12.541	13.246	12.743	13.419
of which PMI	1.999	2.071	2.224	2.456	2.661	2.862
Total	**55.462**	**59.178**	**64.733**	**69.242**	**74.833**	**80.620**

Table 1.2 *Expenditure on health care by source, 1997–2002, as a percentage of total health care expenditure* (Source: *authors' calculations based on figures in Table 1.1 above*)

Expenditure (%)	1997	1998	1999	2000	2001	2002
Public expenditure	80.358	80.354	80.627	80.87	82.971	83.355
Private expenditure,	19.642	19.646	19.373	19.130	17.029	16.645
of which PMI	3.604	3.500	3.436	3.547	3.556	3.550
Total	**100.000**	**100.000**	**100.000**	**100.000**	**100.000**	**100.000**

health care on a privately insured basis to 6.635 million, or to some 11.2% of the population (Laing & Buisson, 2004).

The shift from public–private "sector" to public–private "system"

It is becoming increasingly difficult to identify separate public and private sectors in the United Kingdom's health care system, given the private sector's ability to deliver publicly financed care and the public sector's ability to deliver privately financed care. In today's health care system, the relevant criterion is not the ownership status of the provider, but the function the provider is serving. If the provider is receiving public funds, it is serving a public or NHS function, and if the funds are private, a private market function is being served.

However, given that there remains in place a restriction on flows of funds – that is, a prohibition on the conjoining of public and private revenue streams within a given episode of care – it is still possible to speak of a public "system" (to which access is publicly financed and universal) and a private "system" (to which access is restricted on the basis of willingness to pay). In consequence, despite some form of public–private integration on the delivery side of health care, the system of PMI can still be represented in general terms as providing privately insured access to health care within what continues to be, from the perspective of the PMI subscriber, an entirely separate health care system operating in parallel with the NHS.

Successive governments, including the present one, have stated their commitment to tax-based financing of the NHS. This does not, however, necessarily preclude a widened role for private medical insurers in the evolving health care mix. Recent reform of the United Kingdom health care system can be characterized as follows. Taking as a starting point a relatively integrated NHS (combining insurer, purchaser and provider functions), the government has moved to make the delivery of health care more "independent" – by involving the private sector, by giving NHS providers autonomy (eventually all NHS Trusts will be Foundation Trusts) and by changing the accountability structure, so that providers are accountable to regulators rather than to the Secretary of State for Health (who will no longer answer questions in Parliament relating to Foundation Trusts, referring questioners instead to the regulator). If these reforms succeed, and in coming years there is in place a competitive, independent provider market (facility ownership no longer being of importance), then this leaves the NHS, in effect, as largely an insuring-purchasing organization.

However, debate around reform of NHS purchasing has already begun and it is possible that reform in this area will eventually take a direction similar to reform in the area of health-care provision – namely, towards increased plurality and independence. This scenario is not too distant from the vision touched on in a recent report (Bramley-Harker & Lewis, 2005) endorsed by the Director of Policy at the NHS Confederation and by the former head of the Department of Health's Strategy Unit, which sees a *potential* role for private insurers in a reformed NHS purchasing arena. If this situation does come about, and given the degree of independence that is likely to characterize the health care provider sector at such a time, there is scope not only for private insurers to act as purchasers, or to be otherwise involved in purchasing, for tax-financed patients, but also for the same insurers to introduce restricted packages of supplementary VHI that would cover, for instance, access to better amenities within the context of publicly financed health care. It remains to be seen whether such a situation will indeed transpire and the fundamental separation of public and private revenue streams be weakened. However, given the nature of current debate, this is not an implausible future scenario.

Note on the role of the doctor in the United Kingdom's mixed economy of health

Doctors are at the interface of the public system and the private system, because both systems draw upon the same pool of practitioners. Doctors are free to choose whether to work solely for the NHS, or to take a contract with the NHS that allows them to undertake private practice in their non-NHS time. Where they opt for the latter, the border between their public and private work is policed by the doctors themselves and by their NHS managers. Two important issues arise on the back of this dual-system role: the question of whether NHS care suffers as a result of doctors practising privately (in the form of waiting lists being longer than they might otherwise need to be); and the issue of "queue-jumping", whereby private resources enable the patient to access NHS care more rapidly.

Despite these issues having long been the subject of debate in the United Kingdom, there has been little research on them. On the first question, the single major study, published in 1995, found that private practice was indeed carried out to the detriment of the NHS (Yates, 1995; Yates, 2000). But a more recent study (which did not take into account non-clinical duties, and therefore does not, in effect, provide clear evidence on this particular issue one way or the other) found that surgeons on part-time contracts with the NHS were more productive in their NHS time than those on full-time contracts (Bloor, Maynard & Freemantle, 2004). Nevertheless, as Le Grand has pointed out (Le Grand, 2002):

> the effect of having two systems running alongside one another is to create a perverse incentive structure. A consultant confronted with an NHS patient who needs an operation has an incentive to encourage the patient to 'go private'. For if the patient remains in the NHS, the consultant will have to do the operation without any extra reward, whereas if the patient sees the consultant privately, the consultant will be paid. It is hardly surprising, therefore, that the longest NHS waiting lists occur in the specialities in which specialists have the highest private earnings. If the aim of the policy is to have NHS waiting lists as short as possible, the existence of the private sector running alongside the public service undermines the latter's ability to achieve that aim.

Regarding "queue-jumping", to the best of our knowledge no research has been undertaken, there being instead only anecdotal evidence. The following example illustrates how "queue-jumping" might take place. In the NHS there may be two stages to a waiting list: the first stage would be a preliminary consultation with the specialist, and the second would be the treatment episode. A PMI subscriber who, for instance, faces a high level of cost sharing, might opt for treatment through the NHS but use his/her PMI to access the initial consultation more rapidly, thereby "jumping" part of the queue. In Box 1.1, we provide what we interpret as an illustration of such "queue-jumping", albeit one that is based on out-of-pocket spending rather than PMI. We reproduce the example verbatim from the source in which it appears (a financial intermediary writing about the benefits of self-pay).

Box 1.1 *Faster access to NHS care for private payers* (Source: *Armitage, 2004*)

Carol Richards, a personal assistant in Exeter, cut six months off waiting for treatment by deciding to self-pay. Before receiving treatment, Carol suffered from recurring tonsillitis, usually so severe it would lead to her having to take a week off work.

Her GP put her on a waiting list to see a consultant with a view to having her tonsils removed. Carol was told she faced a six-month wait to see the consultant and another eight months for the operation.

Carol, so fed up with the wait, decided to approach a self-pay specialist. It arranged for Carol to see a consultant at her local hospital within two days, which cost her £95.

The consultant agreed that Carol needed the operation and put her on his waiting list. Although the cost of the operation privately was about £1400, which was more than Carol was able to pay, she was able to cut months off her waiting time.

The NHS consultant contract has recently been changed to provide more incentives for carrying out only NHS work, and to enable better policing of the public–private divide, but it is too early to determine the effect of the new contract on the relationship between public and private systems, as it operates through the doctor.

Chapter 2

Private Medical Insurance: The Product

Basic principles

PMI is a form of traditional indemnity insurance designed to reimburse subscribers for financial loss stemming from the use of health care. (In practice, however, it is common for insurers to reimburse provider facilities directly, though not necessarily the specialist fee component of the charge, thus improving their control over provider charging.) PMI is purchased by individuals, or by employers on their behalf. These alternatives constitute different submarkets, and are referred to here as the individual market and the corporate market, respectively.

The principle that underpins insurance is that groups are better placed to deal with uncertainty than are individuals on their own. Insurance allows an individual to contribute a share of a known group loss – calculable by statisticians and actuaries – in exchange for the security that, should that individual incur a loss, it will be met by the group as a whole. This contribution is called the premium, and, in the case of PMI, is payable monthly or yearly in advance in the individual market (where contracts are for a year, at the end of which they become renewable for further yearly terms), or monthly, yearly or half-yearly in advance in the corporate market (where contracts are renewable on a yearly or half-yearly basis).

For insurance to function, the group loss must be known, but it is imperative that the distribution of this loss across the individuals comprising the group be unknown. When the distribution is unknown, uncertainty is maximized, with all members of the group presenting an equal probability of incurring a higher-than-expected loss or a lower-than-expected loss. Insurance functions to enable the latter to pay for the former (the two balancing each other, in theory, because the overall group loss is known). Insurance has, in consequence, what might be described as a natural tendency to pool "likes", i.e. to group individuals who are similar in terms of their probability of incurring a loss.

If an insurer groups high-risk individuals with low-risk ones, the low-risk individuals will be liable to leave because the distribution of the loss will be less uncertain and the premium they pay will, in part, be functioning as a subsidy to members at higher risk. Low-risk individuals will remain, however, if premiums are adjusted to reflect individual risk, thereby undoing the subsidy made to high-risk individuals, and maximizing uncertainty anew. The principle of actuarial fairness, central to the operation of insurance (Ewald, 1999), refers precisely to this compensatory adjustment of the premium needed to maintain insurance pools intact – allowing them to operate, in effect if not in fact, as pools comprised of "likes".

PMI insurers use two mechanisms to try and achieve actuarial fairness in pricing the product. These mechanisms are underwriting and risk rating (although the latter is usually understood to be part of a wider process of underwriting). They enable insurers to set premiums at rates that reflect the risk the individual brings to the group, and the profitability of an insurer will depend, in part, on its ability to price its products on an actuarially fair basis (or, at any rate, to price them on a more actuarially fair basis than its competitors).

All subscribers to PMI have access to the NHS. If they opt to use their PMI instead of using the NHS, the process begins in the same way. That is, the subscriber will consult his/her GP, who, instead of referring him/her to a consultant within the NHS will refer the individual to a private consultant (who will most probably be an NHS employee working in his/her own non-NHS time). The consultant will set a date for treatment that suits the patient, and, before treatment commences, the patient will usually have to contact his/her PMI insurer to ensure that the proposed treatment and treatment facility are covered by the policy. He/she may also have to contact the insurer at the time of initial referral to ensure that the consultant is on the insurer's list of approved consultants. Following treatment, the private facility will bill the insurer, and the specialist will bill either the insurer or the subscriber (who will then claim reimbursement from the insurer).

The basic product

Some features of PMI are structural and common to all products: rapid access to treatment, a care environment preferable to that available on the NHS, and more choice (of appointment, of doctor, and of provider facility) in comparison with the NHS. The other key shared feature relates to product content, or the core benefits covered. These are defined as "the costs of private treatment for what are commonly known as acute medical conditions" (Association of British Insurers, 2003). PMI also covers items attached to the principal procedure, such as diagnostic tests, nursing, accommodation and outpatient care. However, these associated benefits will usually be limited. The Association of British Insurers' definition of the core PMI benefits is important for three reasons: (i) it names what is common to all products available on the market for PMI; (ii) it is sufficiently vague as to allow substantial product differentiation; and (iii) it highlights the fact that the care financed by PMI is more narrow in scope than the "comprehensive" cover offered by the NHS. This is reflected in the types of procedure for which subscribers commonly use their PMI (see Box 2.1).

There are three basic product templates, which differ according to the degree to which they extend cover beyond these basic or core acute care benefits: comprehensive, standard and budget. Product "options" can be added to the three basic products, and these will either reduce or increase the price of the premium. Product options include extension of cover to dependants, choice regarding depth of coverage (cost sharing), the grade of hospital accommodation permitted, restrictions on choice of hospital, and some incentive items and restrictions on the initiation of PMI-financed care.

In the four decades following the Second World War, the product remained stable around the Association of British Insurers' definition cited above. Then in 1979 there was an important innovation, with PPP healthcare (now AXA PPP) introducing the first reduced-cover, lower-price product designed to appeal to groups not traditionally associated with the purchase of PMI (Laing & Buisson, 2003). Product innovation proceeded in a similar vein from the late 1980s onwards in response to competitive pressures arising from new market entrants, rising aggregate claims expenditure, and a slowdown in the growth of subscriber numbers. With perceived market saturation among the higher-income groups historically associated with the purchase of PMI, product innovation suddenly had to establish new customer bases and function to attract existing customers from other insurers. Although still simple in principle then, PMI has become increasingly complex in reality, with the current proliferation of products making for significant difficulties for product comparison in terms of value for money (see "Regulation and the product" below).

Box 2.1 *Top 20 procedures performed by BUPA hospitals (in alphabetical order)* *(Source: Vallance-Owen, 2004)*

- Autograft bypass of coronary artery(ies)
- Carpal/cubital tunnel release
- Catheterization of right and left sides of heart
- Epidural injection (lumbar)
- Excision of lesion of skin or subcutaneous tissue
- Hysterectomy and removal of uterine adnexae
- Laparoscopic cholecystectomy
- Ligation/stripping of long/short veins
- Phakoemulsification of lens
- Primary repair of inguinal hernia
- Septoplasty of nose
- Sub-acromial decompression
- Surgical removal of impacted teeth
- Thera endo ops cavity of knee
- Thera endo ops semilunar cartilage of knee
- Therapeutic oesophagogastroduodenoscopy
- Tonsillectomy – adult
- Total prosthetic replacement of hip joint
- Total prosthetic replacement of knee joint
- Transurethral resection of the prostate

How private medical insurance is priced

Underwriting

Underwriting is the process by which the insurer decides the nature and amount of risk that it is willing to assume. PMI underwriters usually automatically exclude from cover all pre-existing conditions (i.e. those present at application) – named or otherwise – because of the difficulty of assessing their future cost implications, but at the same time in order to help avert adverse selection, that is, the problem arising from the correlation that exists between the likelihood of needing to make a claim and the propensity to purchase insurance.

Beyond this blanket exclusion, PMI insurers employ two key forms of underwriting. These are full medical underwriting and moratorium underwriting (Association of British Insurers, 2003). They are employed in the individual market and in part of the corporate market only. In the main part of the corporate market, PMI is generally not underwritten (see "Experience rating" below).

Full medical underwriting

Full medical underwriting, also known as medical history declaration, requires the individual to complete a form giving details of his/her medical history and current health status. The insurer may also contact the applicant or the GP for verification or for further information if necessary (British Medical Association, 2002). The questions the insurer asks seek to establish the extent and severity of pre-existing conditions and past conditions and to permit an assessment of the probability of a recurrence, or of a related condition emerging. On the basis of the information provided on the form and by the GP, which will be interpreted in the light of information about the applicant's age and gender, the course of the illness and the treatment received (Chartered Insurance Institute, 2001), the insurer will decide whether a pre-existing or past condition should be excluded and whether to name any other conditions for exclusion which, although they have not appeared in the past, might emerge in the future as a result of the original condition. Pre-existing conditions, past conditions, and potential conditions related to either, will be covered only if the insurer feels that the associated risk is determinable and can be reflected in the premium charged.

Overly strict approaches to full medical underwriting have been widely criticized, including from within the industry itself (which is concerned with unnecessary loss of business). Thus, the Chair of the Association of Medical Insurance Intermediaries describes how underwriting is practised with the example, based on real-world instances that he cites, of an exclusion being imposed on treatment for all skeletal conditions when an applicant mentions an ankle problem – the logic being that the ankle problem could bring about a limp, which might in turn lead to a bad back, which might further lead to a host of other problems. As the commentator notes, "it seems that what we are getting with increasing frequency is not risk assessment, but risk avoidance" (Walker, 2004).

Moratorium underwriting

Moratorium underwriting does not require details of an individual's medical history. Instead, the insurer excludes from cover any condition that existed in the (usually) five years prior to the purchase of PMI, and possibly any directly related conditions that might later emerge. Information about the subscriber's relevant medical history is requested at the time of claim; on the basis of this information, the insurer decides whether or not to meet the claim (moratorium underwriting is also known as point-of-claim underwriting). Excluded conditions become eligible for cover when the subscriber does not experience symptoms or receive treatment, tests or advice for the condition or for related conditions for two full years following the purchase of PMI (Association of British Insurers, 2003). Should symptoms arise – or treatment, tests or advice be given – during this two-year period, the qualifying period of two years starts anew.

Moratorium underwriting is attractive to subscribers because cover commences immediately, because there is no need to complete a medical history declaration, and because conditions that would be permanently excluded under full medical underwriting might come to receive cover under moratorium underwriting if there are no symptoms during the two-year moratorium period. For insurers, it is attractive because of its low administrative burden. There are certain risks associated with moratorium underwriting, however. Consumers may fail to understand what they may or may not make a claim for during the moratorium period (there will usually be more clarity regarding what is excluded from cover under full medical underwriting) and, at worst, consumers may forgo seeking treatment or advice in order to secure cover once the moratorium has come to an end. Consumers may, therefore, incur costs that the insurer will not meet, or they might possibly put their own health at risk (Office of Fair Trading, 1996). Given the risks associated with this type of underwriting, insurers who offer it must offer applicants the option of full medical underwriting too.

Risk rating

If underwriting is concerned with delimiting the risk that the insurer will assume, risk rating is more directly related to the pricing of the risk. The applicant will be assessed primarily by age. Several age bands are used, with different insurers employing different divisions. Risk increases with age, and individuals in higher age bands will accordingly pay higher premiums. Table 2.1 gives an indication of how premiums for PMI rise depending on the band into which the applicant falls.

Insurers argue that risk rating is not an appropriate term to describe how premiums are priced (Comité Européen des Assurances, 1997). They argue that the term community rating is more accurate. Community rating refers to pricing on the basis of the average individual of an insured group – or, alternatively, the known group loss divided by the number comprising the group. In the PMI market, community rating exists in so far as the value accorded to each age band reflects the average for all members of that band across the population as a whole. However, the division of age into different bands means that individuals can be rated on an individual basis, so that the most that can be said in defence of the position that there is no risk rating is that risk rating rests – as, almost inevitably, it must – on community rating

Table 2.1 *Average indexed premium, by age* (Source: *Association of British Insurers,* *2003*)

Age	Indexed premium (%)
35	100
40	116
45	125
50	148
55	161
60	208
65	268

across the population as a whole. In other words, if all 40-year-olds pay the same premium, they are nevertheless rated first as 40-year-olds and "priced" accordingly.

Most insurers place a ceiling on the age at which new applicants can be accepted: 65, 74 or 75 (*Cover*, 2004a). As with pre-existing conditions, this is because when a given age is reached, insurers find it difficult to determine an appropriate price for the premium (particularly as the probability of loss is approaching 100%, at which point insurance ceases to function).

In practice, insurers use other risk categories too. For example, they may employ information about an applicant's gender, occupational status, smoking status and place of residence (by postcode) to calculate the premium. Gender, occupational and smoking status all work in the same way as age, in that the value accorded a nonsmoker, for instance, or a worker in a particular industry, or a woman, will be calculated on the basis of information derived from the category across the whole population. Place of residence differs as a risk factor, in that it attempts to capture elements such as local population size, local NHS facilities per head, local NHS waiting times, and the price attached to private facilities locally (Chartered Insurance Institute, 2001).

Recently, insurers have been introducing further risk categories. AXA PPP, for example, has introduced what it terms "Personally Designated Quotations", which use information on the applicant's height and weight in assessing the risk presented (*Cover*, 2003; *Insurance Age*, 2003). However, in this instance the provision of the information is entirely voluntary – which means that it represents an attempt to attract customers who would benefit from providing it, that is, those at low risk of incurring a loss (at least as measured by height and weight). This, then, is a form of market segmentation on the back of product design, or, in effect, a type of risk selection. It enables low risks to signal their risk status more effectively and thus to reduce the subsidy made to individuals at higher risk that their contributions continue to incorporate given the community underpinnings of risk-band valuation (and, at the same time, of course, serving to attract customers from competing insurers under whom low risks are unable to signal their risk status so effectively).

In the individual market, there is guaranteed renewal of the policy at the end of the contract year, with the premium being adjusted only to reflect the previous year's (if higher than anticipated) expected changes in aggregate claims expenditure across the insured pool, general and medical inflation, and changes in the loading charge (see "Further dimensions of price" below). The premium will also be adjusted to reflect the subscriber's move into a new age band, but other than in relation to the category of age, there is no further risk rating or underwriting at the point of renewal (thus, if the subscriber has suffered from medical conditions and made claims in the preceding contract year, the price at the renewal stage will not try to capture this).

Although there is no significant risk rating at the point of renewal, in both markets the benefits covered by the policy may change (in the corporate market this will usually apply at the level of the individual rather than that of the group as a whole) without this being reflected in the price of the premium. For instance, PMI cover for a given medical condition might be withdrawn if treatment has exceeded a certain time period or if the condition has become chronic (that is, is no longer amenable to care designed to be applied to acute conditions).

Experience rating

The corporate market is divided into small-group schemes (usually employee groups of fewer than 50) and large-group schemes (groups of over 50). Small-group schemes are generally underwritten and priced in a similar way to that used in the individual market, but will take account of claims history, group size and age composition, type of industry and company location. Large-group schemes, in contrast, tend not to be underwritten but are priced solely on the basis of the group's claims experience for the previous year. Experience rating in the corporate market is often thought of as a form of community rating, as all employees within the group will be accorded the same risk value (i.e. the average for the group). However, experience rating can equally be thought of as a form of risk rating, as it is the single employer who pays the premium (even if it is those who are covered who are referred to as the subscribers), and past claims expenditure is, in effect, a reflection of the risk presented by the group as a single entity.

Large-group schemes require cover to be extended to all employees within given categories such as age group, status within the company, and length of service. This is to ensure that risk is spread widely, and that adverse selection is avoided. Renewal of group schemes rests with the insurer, so there is no guarantee of cover being extended into subsequent years. At the point of renewal, which will take place either yearly or half-yearly, the insurer might alter the terms of the contract or refuse to renew if the claims experience is sufficiently adverse. A group with light claims experience can expect to see an allowance in the cost of cover for the coming year or half-year (Chartered Insurance Institute, 2001; Organisation for Economic Co-operation and Development, 2001).

Although, in the absence of underwriting, large-group schemes do not exclude pre-existing conditions (except in some marginal instances), employers are able to exert significant control over product design, and may request exclusions of particular pre-existing conditions – this will usually involve mental illnesses or addiction – in order to lower the price of the premium. In a survey of employers, AON Health Solutions found that from 1999 to 2000, 23.7% excluded cover for some pre-existing conditions, and that in 2001 this had risen to 44.9% of employers (AON Health Solutions, 2002).

Further dimensions of price

There are four dimensions of price. The first relates to the scope of cover purchased after any underwriting (see "The three product categories" below). The second relates to the risk characteristics of the purchaser. These two dimensions are fundamental, and the price of the premium will always reflect a combination of the two – that is to say, there is no single price for a given level of cover that applies equally to all in an actuarially fair market (or a market that aspires to being actuarially fair) comprised of individuals who are non-alike across the dimensions that matter.

The third dimension of price relates to what we refer to as product options (see "Product options" below). When the basic product has been chosen, the subscriber may choose to reduce the price by accepting constraints on the way in which he/she uses the PMI. Constraints on use will reduce the insurer's claims-related expenditure, and it is this reduction that will be reflected in the lower price of the premium. The subscriber might also increase the price of the premium by, for instance, choosing to extend cover to dependants.

The fourth dimension is the "loading charge". This reflects the insurer's administrative costs and profit. It also reflects insurance premium tax, currently set at 5% of the premium. In the perfectly competitive market, where information is complete and symmetrical between consumers and producers, insurers compete on the basis of this charge alone. However, in common with many other insurance markets, the PMI market is characterized by significant information problems, and competition does not operate on the basis of the loading charge alone.

The three product categories

Insurers generally use three categories to describe PMI products: comprehensive, standard and budget. These descriptors refer only to the scope of coverage, and, in particular, to the scope of coverage offered beyond the acute-care benefits covered by all PMI products. They do not, therefore, refer to the presence or absence of any of the product options mentioned above.

Comprehensive policies

Comprehensive policies offer the widest range of benefits and are the most expensive to purchase. Beyond the core benefits, they offer a significant level of outpatient care and access to a wide range of further benefits. The term "comprehensive" may be misleading, however, as these policies might restrict cover for certain types of care to monthly or annual monetary amounts and, moreover, as the medical director of AXA PPP has remarked, "none of the PMI companies aim to provide comprehensive health cover" (cited in Seib, 2004). The benefits offered under comprehensive policies will vary by insurer, but will probably include items from among those listed in Box 2.2.

Standard policies

Standard policies offer fewer benefits beyond the core benefits, but are cheaper to purchase. They will not usually provide cover for psychiatric treatment, for complications arising from pregnancy and childbirth, or for services such as repatriation, optical care and private ambulance services. Standard policies may also automatically incorporate a restriction on choice of hospital and a monetary limit on outpatient benefits, or alternatively limit these to care relating directly to an inpatient or day-patient episode (Chartered Insurance Institute, 2001). They may, however, offer cash incentives for subscribers to seek care with the NHS rather than through their PMI policies.

Budget policies

Budget policies are the least expensive. These enable consumers to purchase a relatively limited quantity of cover for a significantly lower premium. Some budget policies will restrict cover to the more important or expensive types of treatment, including most types of inpatient and day care, but most place automatic restrictions on the choice of hospital or the level of hospital accommodation permitted. The more restrictive budget policies focus on providing cover for

Box 2.2 *Benefits beyond acute care benefits under comprehensive products* (Sources: *Chartered Insurance Institute, 2001; CareHealth, 2004*)

- Treatment for mental and addictive illnesses, with the exception of alcohol and/or drug abuse
- Repatriation to the United Kingdom in the event of a medical emergency, or the provision of private medical cover while overseas
- Treatment of complications arising from pregnancy and childbirth
- Complementary and alternative medical treatment
- Dental treatment provided by a specialist up to an annual monetary limit
- Optical care up to an annual monetary limit
- A cash payment if treatment is received as an NHS patient rather than as a private patient
- A cash payment for each night spent as an NHS inpatient, usually set as a given amount per night
- Provision of a guest room for a parent to accompany a child during an inpatient stay
- Home nursing services
- Private ambulance services

areas in which NHS performance is perceived to be especially wanting, and some limit care to that which cannot be provided by the NHS within six weeks following diagnosis by a consultant (the so-called six-week policies).

Industry commentators note that although the best standard policies offer good value for money, many can be over-complicated and require professional advice. They also note that six-week policies offer poor value for money, are expensive for the service they provide, and rarely live up to consumer expectations (Private Health Partnership, 2004). Budget policies, like comprehensive policies, can be complex products, and it has been pointed out that consumers might easily fail to appreciate the degree to which the scope of cover that budget products offer is limited (Chartered Insurance Institute, 2001).

Items excluded from cover

There are some items of health care to which cover is usually not extended under any of the product categories. These are referred to as standard or general exclusions. Some relate to chronic conditions and some relate to predictable forms of health care use, such as GP services, preventive treatment, general pregnancy-related care and care relating to pre-existing conditions. General exclusions exist largely to avert the emergence of adverse selection and moral hazard problems, but they also exist to protect the insurer against catastrophic loss (individual claims probabilities have to be independent of one another, and insurers will withdraw cover from claims that are not independent – that is, those resulting from a single causal factor such as war or mass accident). Cover for accident and emergency care is also excluded, as it is high-cost and, moreover, is provided solely by the NHS. Box 2.3 provides a more detailed list.

The range of exclusions has changed over time as new technologies have emerged and in response to cost pressures faced by the industry as a whole. Two recent restrictions of cover have been controversial: exclusion of caesarean sections and exclusion of mental health problems. In 2001, AXA PPP stopped offering cover for caesarean sections because it was finding it difficult to distinguish those conducted for medical reasons from those carried out on an elective basis. Given that some 50% of deliveries in private hospitals are by caesarean section, compared to a national average of 20%, the insurer felt that this growing trend towards caesarean sections was not financially sustainable (Laing & Buisson, 2003).

Mental health is another area in which PMI cover has been increasingly restricted over time. This is because of the complex and long-term nature of mental health treatment and the difficulties in differentiating between acute and non-acute care in this area. In 2003, for example, Western Provident Association (WPA) stopped offering cover for mental health in the individual market (Laing & Buisson, 2003). Notably, however, the AON Health Solutions survey found that only 36.8% of employers restricted psychiatric benefits in 2001, a figure that was down from 44.4% in 1999/2000 and 44.0% in 1998 (this does not include the exclusion of mental health problems under the heading of pre-existing conditions). It is possible that employers are now less likely to restrict psychiatric benefits, because of greater awareness of employer liability with respect to mental health and work-related stress (AON Health Solutions, 2002).

Viewed from a different angle, the exclusion of pre-existing conditions can lead to what might be termed a sticky market problem. If the subscriber is receiving care for a particular condition under his/her current insurer, the incentives built into the system are for the subscriber to remain with that insurer, despite the existence of a more highly valued product elsewhere, as switching to another insurer will mean that the condition in question will be excluded from cover as a pre-existing one. This stickiness – the way the system works to prevent ill subscribers from joining new insurers – works to defend insurers from adverse selection problems, but means that the choices faced by the consumer have been severely constrained.

Box 2.3 *General PMI exclusions (Source: Chartered Insurance Institute, 2001)*

- Pre-existing conditions
- Mental and addictive conditions and disorders (although some insurers will cover treatment on a discretionary basis)
- Pregnancy and childbirth (if a caesarean section is deemed medically necessary, the insurer might cover the cost, but only on a discretionary basis)
- Contraception, assisted reproduction, sterilization, sexual dysfunction, or termination of pregnancy
- Treatment for, or resulting from, acquired immunodeficiency syndrome or infection with human immunodeficiency virus
- Unproven or experimental treatment
- Surgery intended to improve a person's appearance and/or which is undertaken for the purpose of removing body tissue that is not diseased (though insurers will make discretionary benefit payments to subscribers who require surgery to restore disfigurement as a result of accident or disease)
- Treatment for illness or injury resulting from nuclear or chemical contamination, war, invasion, acts of foreign enemies, hostilities (whether war be declared or not), civil war, rebellion, revolution, insurrection or military or usurped power
- Renal dialysis (some insurers may cover renal dialysis if it is needed for the immediate purpose of kidney transplantation or in connection with immediate management of acute secondary renal failure)
- Treatment intended to relieve conditions associated with bodily change which arise from physiological or natural causes such as hormone replacement therapy linked to ageing
- Treatment provided by an individual who is not recognized as a specialist by the insurer
- Dental or oral surgery
- Treatment of chronic conditions (other than acute episodes)

Clarity regarding coverage

The precise scope of cover provided by a PMI product can be unclear, as it will rest on the interpretation of important terms such as "acute", "chronic", "pre-existing", "short-term treatment", "long-term treatment" and "medically necessary". Prior to the GISC's introduction of Practice Requirement E2 (see "Self-regulation under the General Insurance Standards Council" below), there were no industry-wide definitions of the most important of these terms, and most insurers used their own (Office of Fair Trading, 1996).

This is reflected in the evolution of the principal guide to buying PMI, *Are you buying Private Medical Insurance?* (Association of British Insurers, 2003). Earlier editions did not define "acute condition", but the latest edition adopts the definition given by the GISC: "a disease, illness or injury that is likely to respond quickly to treatment which aims to return you to the state of health you were in immediately before suffering the disease, illness or injury, or which leads to your full recovery" (General Insurance Standards Council, 2003; Association of British Insurers, 2003).

For "pre-existing condition", there are several definitions available:

- an illness or physical condition already diagnosed or treated prior to PMI cover commencing (Chartered Insurance Institute, 2001);

- an illness from which you are already suffering or which you have already had (Association of British Insurers, 2003);

- an illness or medical problem you had before joining an insurance scheme even though you may not have received treatment for it (Charitable Hospitals Federation, not dated);

- any disease, illness or injury for which you have received medication, advice or treatment, or you have experienced symptoms, whether the condition has been diagnosed or not in the *xxx* years before the start of your cover (the same period is not common to all insurers) (General Insurance Standards Council, 2003).

The first two definitions are substantially different from the second two, in that they imply that the condition will have been diagnosed or treated and, therefore, be known to the individual concerned. In contrast, the third and fourth definitions imply that cover would be excluded even if the individual were not aware that he or she had suffered from an illness or injury in the past, which is likely to give rise to confusion or possible conflict at the point of claim. Unlike the first three, the GISC definition also suggests that the timing of the illness suffered is relevant.

Chronic conditions

Regarding the term "chronic condition", the GISC defines this as a disease, illness or injury that has one of the following characteristics:

- it continues indefinitely and has no known cure

- it comes back or is likely to come back

- it is permanent

- you need to be rehabilitated or specially trained to cope with it

- it needs long-term monitoring, consultations, check-ups, examinations or tests.

In addition to recommending that this definition be used by insurers, GISC rules state that, where appropriate, a "chronic condition explanation" should be provided prior to customers committing to purchasing PMI. This should include an introductory paragraph based on the following headings:

- what is a chronic condition?

- what does this mean in practice?

- what if your condition gets worse?

- examples of chronic conditions.

Despite these attempts to foster clarity, recent research by the charity CancerBACUP has highlighted disagreement among insurers about whether conditions are chronic or acute in nature. In the CancerBACUP study, 14 insurers were asked whether subscribers who develop cancer would be covered for treatment throughout the entire course of their illness. Responses from the eight insurers who replied show that not all insurers cover cancer treatment for its entire course. Some stop covering cancer care once the cancer becomes palliative or the condition chronic, while others will provide cover for "active treatment" or "acute flare-ups" (CancerBACUP, 2004). Importantly, what the responding insurers did not say was how they define palliative care, what they mean by active treatment and acute flare-ups, at what point cancer is considered to become chronic and whether policies cover treatment when the goal is to slow the progression of the disease or improve quality of life rather than to cure.

Product options

Once individuals have chosen the level of cover they require, they can select further options, which will affect the price. These include:

- restrictions on choice of hospital

- level of hospital accommodation permitted

- depth of coverage (level of cost sharing)

- application of a no-claims discount.

These options are taken up differently in the different submarkets. In the corporate market, the scope of cover offered is fairly standard throughout, but there is wide variation in terms of cost sharing options and restrictions on treatment facilities (Incomes Data Services, 2003). These two options are also popular in the individual market, but here the use of incentive items (such as no-claims discounts and cash payments for using the NHS instead of PMI) and restrictions on initiating the use of PMI (for example, the so-called six-week policies) are far more common than in the corporate market.

Hospital networks

In the second half of the 1990s, insurers began to introduce hospital network options. These would provide subscribers with a reduced premium in exchange for accepting a restriction on their choice of hospital to those with which the insurer had been able to negotiate a discount. BUPA was the first insurer to introduce this option, and was quickly followed by others. Network size has increased significantly since, with the larger insurers having hospitals in all areas.

Industry analysts report that, in the late 1990s, network take-up in the individual market was rapid, but that it had begun to level out by 1999. At that point, take-up began to grow in the corporate market, however, with over half (Laing & Buisson, 2003), or some 63% (AON Health Solutions, 2002), of all corporate PMI schemes having selected the network option by 2002.

For providers, the reason for belonging to a network lies in the promise of increased business vis-à-vis the alternative situation of not belonging to a network – but at the cost of having to discount standard prices. BUPA, notably, does not provide hospitals in its network (or other hospitals from whom it has obtained a discount) with a guarantee of business volume (Competition Commission, 2000). The fact that hospitals are willing, or feel it necessary, to proceed on this basis is an indication of this insurer's market power.

Hospital networks usually concentrate on including hospitals belonging to the hospital groups, with private patient units and independent (non-group) hospitals being included only in areas where there is no group hospital available. Given the nationwide reach of the hospital groups, this has been one of the key factors driving the purchase or closure of many independent hospitals, unable as they are to attract a sufficient volume of PMI-generated business when located in the vicinity of a group hospital.

The introduction of the network option has had another significant effect – namely the phenomenon of "consultant drag". For reasons of convenience, consultants choose to treat all their patients (network and non-network alike) in the hospital in which they are obliged to treat their network patients. Consequently, by reinforcing the dominance of the major hospital groups, "consultant drag" again presents a threat to hospitals not included in a network (Competition Commission, 2000).

The number of hospitals in a network (or networks, as insurers may offer more than one list, reflecting the different levels of discount that have been obtained) varies by insurer. Although there may be risk attached to the network option when the decision to include a hospital has been driven by financial reasons alone (Chartered Insurance Institute, 2001), the OFT found in 1999 that network options had been successful in encouraging hospitals to compete on price and quality, and therefore worked to the benefit of the consumer (Office of Fair Trading, 1999).

Hospital accommodation

The major insurers all offer an option regarding the level of hospital accommodation to which the subscriber will have access. The level of comfort offered for each band of accommodation will differ from hospital to hospital, depending on the prices the hospital charges. Thus, for example, a Band 3 level of accommodation may provide access to a private room with en suite bathroom in one hospital, but in another, more expensive hospital it may provide access to a similar room without the bathroom.

Cost sharing

Cost sharing options in the form of co-insurance are more common in the corporate market than in the individual market. Co-insurance requires the subscriber to pay a proportion of the cost of any claim, but perhaps up to a specified limit only – for example, 10% of all costs up to an annual limit of £2000 per person covered by the policy (Chartered Insurance Institute, 2001). The insurer WPA currently leads in the development of co-insurance policies – which it terms "shared responsibility" – in both the corporate market and the individual market.

Excesses are a more widespread form of cost sharing across both markets. An excess is the amount a subscriber has to pay towards the cost of any claim (for example, the first £100), with the insurer paying the balance. Most PMI products now include the excess option, which may apply per claim or per policy year. Policies with excesses are designed to appeal to younger people, who are less likely to require treatment but want to be insured against serious conditions, and to lower-income customers who may be attracted by the lower premium price (Laing & Buisson, 2003).

The AON Health Solutions survey found that, in 2001, 36.5% of employers operated an excess, up from 33.9% in 2000 and 27.0% in 1998 (AON Health Solutions, 2002). A subsequent survey found that this proportion had risen to 39.6% in 2002–2003, and to 43.5% in 2003–2004 (AON Consulting, 2004). Excesses are, in principle, not popular with employers, as employees perceive them to represent a lower level of cover. But, in the face of rising premiums, the excess is one way of keeping the costs of premiums and claims down. The most popular excess level in the corporate market is between £51 and £100 (AON Health Solutions, 2002).

Typical excess amounts are relatively low, ranging from £50 to £500. Recently, some insurers have developed so-called high-excess policies offering substantially reduced premiums in exchange for excesses ranging from £1000 to £5000. Such policies place considerable financial risk on the subscriber, but savings on the premium can be high (CareHealth, 2004).

Although corporate PMI is employer-purchased, employers may decide to have the employee contribute to the cost of the premium. According to the AON Consulting survey, however, only 12.5% of employers choose to do this (AON Consulting, 2004). Where an employee contribution is required, this might be considered a form of cost sharing, but it is one that pertains more strictly to the product structure rather than to the category of product options.

No-claims discount

No-claims discounts are currently offered by two insurers: AXA PPP and Standard Life Healthcare (CareHealth, 2004). These discounts reward policy-holders who do not claim, and can result in significant cost savings over long periods. However, policies with no-claims discounts might be confusing for consumers, who might not fully understand what will happen to their premiums should they require treatment and make a claim, and who might risk forgoing care (or PMI-financed care) so as to maintain the discount on their premium. Moreover, publicity matter can be misleading in terms of the precise nature of the saving made through this option (CareHealth, 2004).

Regulation and the product

The Office of Fair Trading investigations into private medical insurance

In the United Kingdom market (unlike the VHI markets of some other countries; Mossialos & Thomson, 2004), there is no regulation of the product and the pricing. Formal regulation in the United Kingdom is limited, rather, to financial or prudential regulation of insurance companies, with a focus on securing company solvency. However, regulatory pressures have been applied with respect to the PMI product in the past (resulting in more stringent industry self-regulation), and new statutory regulation of insurance sales that came into effect in January 2005 may have some indirect material impact on product design and pricing.

The OFT is the United Kingdom's regulatory agency for consumer protection. In the second half of the 1990s, the OFT – prompted by concern relating to information-related consumer detriment within the market for PMI (see, for example, Calnan, Cant & Grabe, 1993; Youngman, 1994) – launched two investigations. These focused only on the individual market, as consumer vulnerability was perceived to be higher there than in the corporate market. The resulting two reports identified serious problems regarding the product, and were critical of industry practices.

The first report highlighted three core areas of concern. The first related to the ability of consumers to compare different products: "different plans are presented in different ways, and it is difficult – if not impossible for those outside the industry – to compare them in terms of value for money". In particular, the OFT felt that individual insurers had deliberately developed their own preferred terminology to make their products difficult to compare with those of their competitors. The second area of concern related to moratorium underwriting, the report noting that "exclusions may well not come to light until a claim is made, making it impossible to judge whether a particular policy offers value for money". Moreover, under moratorium underwriting, "consumers are given a clear incentive not to seek medical advice during the moratorium period". The third problem related to the absence of information regarding past and likely future increases in the premium (Office of Fair Trading, 1996).

In this first report, the OFT made several recommendations. These included that products be presented in a common format and in clear language, and that a "benchmark" or "core terms" approach be developed to enable straightforward comparison among products. In relation to moratorium underwriting, the OFT recommended that this practice should be abandoned. Finally, regarding increases in the price of premiums, the OFT suggested that information should be provided on why prices rise and how prices have risen in the past, and a projection should be given of how they might rise in the future (Office of Fair Trading, 1996).

In 1997, the Association of British Insurers responded, assuring the OFT that it would address the problem of product comparability, but criticizing it for being overly harsh with respect to moratorium underwriting. It also noted that product proliferation could be explained on the basis of competition within the industry, and that the introduction of a "benchmark product" to aid comparability would have a "restrictive effect, stifling product innovation" (reported in Office of Fair Trading, 1998a).

The OFT continued to monitor the industry during this period, and in a second report found its response wanting (Office of Fair Trading, 1998a). The press release accompanying the second report was entitled *Final Warning to Health Insurers,* and in it the Director General of Fair Trading, referring to the industry response to the earlier report as "dismal", threatened comprehensive regulatory action (Office of Fair Trading, 1998b).

This second report gave more detailed recommendations regarding product presentation, attaching a separate document called *Core Term Products* (Office of Fair Trading, 1998c), which provided a template for insurers to follow that would facilitate product comparison. The report also stated that the practice of moratorium underwriting need not be discontinued if new OFT guidance were followed, i.e. if moratorium underwriting were to be accompanied by oral and written explanations of how it functions and if emphasis was given to the advisability of not forgoing medical advice during the moratorium period. The report also recommended that the sales process be monitored to ensure that these recommendations were being adhered to (Office of Fair Trading, 1998a).

In a press release in 2000 (without any further report), the OFT noted that the industry had improved its literature with respect to product information and that consumers were now better able to compare products across insurers. As some commentators noted, however, it is not "clear how far this statement was based on evidence that consumers could actually compare products in practice. It appears that the OFT was exercising its own judgement and assuming that comparison would be easier based on the existence of new sales literature" (Keen, Light & Mays, 2001). On the other issues of central concern, the OFT was less accommodating, noting that "vague warnings about the escalating cost of premiums and the conditions attached to moratorium-based policies do not address all our concerns and we will continue to press … for improvements" (Office of Fair Trading, 2000).

Self-regulation under the General Insurance Standards Council

In 2000, there was a major industry development with the establishment of GISC, the insurance industry's self-regulating body (self-regulation had formerly been carried out under the auspices of the Association of British Insurers, which functioned at the same time as the industry's representative body). GISC was set up as an independent, non-statutory body with responsibility for regulating sales, marketing and service standards in all areas of general insurance. Its remit was also to ensure fair treatment for customers. All the major PMI insurers and intermediaries were members of GISC, and as such they were bound by GISC's General Insurance Code (relating to private customers) and the Commercial Code (relating to commercial customers). They were also bound by any relevant Practice Requirements.

GISC was particularly active in the area of PMI. In 2003, it began to develop a Practice Requirement for PMI, following consultation with industry stakeholders, that would become effective from January 2004. This Practice Requirement (now no longer available; see Box 2.4 for the main text) was binding on all GISC members providing PMI-related information and services to existing or potential customers. The Practice Requirement partially addresses the key problems highlighted by the OFT, barring the premium-projection requirement. The main text incorporates the later OFT recommendations on moratorium underwriting, and a core benefits table to be included in the "key information" section of the product literature is provided in an appendix (reproduced here in Box 2.5).

In 2001, the government announced that general insurance sales, including the sale of PMI, would come under the statutory regulation of the FSA, as of 14 January 2005, and that GISC would consequently be disbanded (HM Treasury, 2001). GISC has now been disbanded, and its web site refers visitors to the FSA web site.

To the best of our knowledge, there has been no independent assessment of the degree to which PMI insurers complied with the Practice Requirement in the year following its introduction. Replacement of self-regulation by GISC with external regulation by the FSA means that Practice Requirement E2 is now redundant. Nevertheless, the FSA shares with GISC a desire to ensure that consumers are given clear information prior to sale, and at the point of sale, and in this sense the FSA represents continuity rather than change regarding the process initiated by GISC.

Regulation by the Financial Services Authority

Responsibility for the regulation of insurance sales, including sales of PMI, now rests with the FSA. This is the first time that insurance selling and administration has been subject to external statutory regulation, and insurers and intermediaries must comply with FSA rules or they will be committing a criminal offence (Financial Services Authority, 2003). The relevant rules are set out in the book *Insurance: Conduct of Business* (Financial Services Authority, 2004a).

Box 2.4 *Practice Requirement E2 – Private Medical Insurance* (Source: *General Insurance Standards Council, 2003*)

1 This Practice Requirement describes requirements and guidance for Members who wish to provide Private Medical Insurance (PMI), General Insurance Activity-related information or services to their Private Customers and potential Private Customers.

Matching customer requirements

2 Members must make sure, as far as possible, that a Private Customer who purchases a PMI policy understands its main features and that the policy being purchased is appropriate to their needs.

3 Members must, as far as possible, obtain the following relevant information from Private Customers:

3.1 their current and recent medical history;

3.2 details of any cover held under an existing medical insurance or eligibility for company benefits;

3.3 their hospital requirements; and

3.4 any specific requirements.

Information about products and services

4 All potential Private Customers must be given a copy of the Association of British Insurers' consumer guide to PMI, Are You Buying Private Medical Insurance?

5 Members must include prescribed Key Product Information as part of their marketing and sales literature, in accordance with the Guidelines for providing Key Product Information for PMI Customers in Appendix 6.

6 Private Customers and potential Private Customers must be provided with the following information before they make a final commitment to buy their insurance:

6.1 why a policy, or policies are being proposed (and a comparison of price, cover and/or service where a choice of more than one product is being offered);

6.2 the benefits available under the policy and any significant or unusual medical or other exclusions or restrictions applying which are included in, and imposed by, the standard terms and conditions;

6.3 an explanation of the principles of medical underwriting, stressing the need for the Private Customer to give full information in response to any questions asked;

6.4 where relevant, a Chronic Condition Explanation in the format contained in Appendix 9;

6.5 an explanation of the restrictions that may apply to the treatment of pre-existing and chronic conditions;

(cont.)

6.6 details of the implications of switching their cover from one Insurer to another Insurer on a similar or a different product;

6.7 the implications of reducing or changing cover with the same Insurer;

6.8 details of any excess available, how this affects the premium and operates when a claim is made; and

6.9 any restrictions on hospitals and consultants as a result of any hospital networks or agreements.

7 If a moratorium product is being offered to a Private Customer, the Private Customer must receive a full and clear explanation that:

7.1 any pre-existing and related conditions will not be covered for an initial period;

7.2 any such condition may become eligible for cover only when there has been a continuous period, stipulated by the Insurer, during which time there has not been treatment, symptoms, medication, tests and/or advice for that condition (or a related one). Private Customers must be advised not to forgo medical treatment in order to achieve this;

7.3 chronic and long term conditions which require treatment and/or monitoring, are not likely to be eligible for cover because of the need to remain free of treatment, symptoms, medication, tests and advice; and

7.4 full medical underwriting is available as an alternative.

8 Members must also provide any other information required by the Private Customer Code to be given to Private Customers before they make a final commitment to buy their insurance.

Advice and recommendations

9 Members will only discuss or advise on matters of which they have knowledge. As a minimum, Employees who are advising on, or selling, PMI must have knowledge and understanding of the following:

9.1 the general principles of PMI underwriting, and how different methods can affect Private Customers at the claims stage;

9.2 the implications involved in transferring PMI cover from one provider to another; and

9.3 awareness of other health-related insurance, including cash plans, income protection and critical illness insurance.

Confirming your cover

10 As soon as possible after cover has commenced and before any "cooling-off" period finishes, Private Customers will be given a full and clear explanation of the following (unless this information has already been provided):

(cont.)

10.1 a full list of general exclusions which apply to the policy;

10.2 the fact that the Insurer does have the right to change the terms;

10.3 that the Private Customer has the right to renew cover but only on the terms and conditions generally offered by the Insurer at the renewal date;

10.4 that premiums generally rise above the rate of inflation on renewal and that there may be other factors which directly affect premiums, such as age and any no-claims discount;

10.5 the arrangements for making and paying claims, including whether payment is made directly to the provider of services or to the insured person;

10.6 any underwriting terms on pre-existing medical conditions or conditions which will apply including where the Private Customer is transferring cover from a previous PMI policy.

Documentation

11 Where a Member uses a word or phrase that is defined in Appendix 8 in policy or other documents then that Member must use the common definition.

The government's decision to extend external regulation to the sale of insurance was mainly prompted by the legal requirement to incorporate Directive 2002/92/EC of December 2002 on Insurance Mediation – the Insurance Mediation Directive – into United Kingdom law (European Commission, 2003). The Insurance Mediation Directive deals specifically with enabling intermediaries to operate across national borders, but the United Kingdom Government decided to extend the provisions it contained to all insurance sales. The Insurance Mediation Directive represented an opportunity for the government to extend regulation in the insurance industry, but extending it was also a matter of ensuring a level playing field between insurers and intermediaries with respect to insurance sales, with neither being disadvantaged with respect to the other by the presence or absence of formal regulation.

FSA rules apply to all areas of sales and administration, including the use of financial promotions, claims handling, policy cancellation and the distance-selling of insurance. Of relevance here are the two items headed "Suitability" and "Product disclosure". The former relates to ensuring that the policy is the appropriate one for the customer, and that a statement of the agreed "demands and needs" of the customer be provided in a durable medium. Under "Suitability", the agent must ensure "that cover is sufficient for the risks the customer wants to insure", taking into account "any relevant exclusions or conditions in the contract" and taking into account the cost of the contract (Financial Services Authority, 2004b).

Box 2.5 *Core benefits table* (Source: *General Insurance Standards Council, 2003*)

Benefits	Cover available	Notes
Inpatient and day-patient treatment		
Hospital charges		
Consultants'/specialists' fees		
Diagnostic tests		
Radiotherapy/chemotherapy		
Psychiatric treatment		
Outpatient treatment		
Consultations with a consultant/specialist		
Diagnostic tests		
Radiotherapy/chemotherapy		
Physiotherapy		
Psychiatric treatment		
Additional Benefits		
Nursing at home		
Private ambulance		
Parent accommodation when staying with a child covered by the policy		
NHS cash benefit		

Notes on the use of the prescribed Core Benefits Table:

1 Where there is no limit, this should be indicated by a tick.

2 When limits apply, these must be indicated on the table.

3 When a benefit is not available, this should be indicated by a cross.

4 When qualifying criteria apply, these should be referred to in the "Notes" column.

"Product disclosure" relates to the provision of information about the product, and sets out what information must be provided and how it is to be provided. In the individual market, the customer must be given, among other items and "in good time before the conclusion of a contract", a "Policy Summary". This must be "in a prominent place within the other documents and clearly identifiable as key information that the retail customer should read", and must also be "separate from the other content of the document in which it is included". The FSA states that the summary "is not intended to communicate the full terms and conditions" of the contract, but must "properly describe the contract" without overloading the customer with detail.

The FSA's template for the Policy Summary incorporates 13 headings, two being "significant features and benefits" and "significant and unusual exclusions or limitations". The FSA handbook defines "significant and unusual exclusion" as an exclusion "that would tend to affect the decision … to buy", and provides the following examples (Financial Services Authority, 2004a):

- for non-investment insurance contracts that are pure protection contracts or medical insurance: deferred payment periods; exclusion of certain conditions or diseases; exclusion of pre-existing medical conditions; and moratorium periods;

- for all types of non-investment insurance contracts: limits on the amounts of cover; limits on the period for which benefits will be paid; restrictions on eligibility to claim such as age or employment status; and excesses.

The FSA also requires that the customer "be told orally of the importance of reading the policy summary, especially the section on significant and unusual exclusions" (Financial Services Authority, 2004b).

Neither the OFT, GISC, nor the FSA sought powers to regulate the PMI product directly – something that has now been prohibited in markets for supplementary VHI by European legislation (Mossialos & Thomson, 2004). Instead, they focused their regulatory efforts on PMI sales. The concern shared by all three was that the nature of competition in the market for PMI disadvantaged consumers vis-à-vis providers of PMI. In the market for PMI, there is no "common product" to which a price is subsequently attached, with insurers competing to provide the same product at the lowest price – despite the development of the core benefits table as an aid to comparison. This is partly because of the nature of product pricing in this market, where price reflects both product content and purchaser characteristics (to which different insurers will accord different values). However, it also has to do with the product proliferation that characterizes this market, with insurers competing on the basis of product differentiation (product competition or, strictly, product–price competition) rather than on the basis of price and quality alone.

Thus – in a case highlighted by CareHealth – BUPA, for instance, offers 3960 alternative choices for one of its products, each impacting on the final price. There are five core variants of the product, three options for hospitals covered, three options for premium rates (standard, fixed over five years, or fixed over ten years), eight excess levels and eleven options for additional cover – meaning that an individual must choose from 3960 alternative product designs. BUPA presents an extreme case, but the range of options facing a 50-year-old man looking at other insurers is also high, at 114 for AXA PPP, 48 for Standard Life Healthcare and 44 for Norwich Union Healthcare (CareHealth, 2004).

Once purchaser characteristics have been incorporated into price, product comparison in terms of value for money may become virtually impossible within any time constraint considered reasonable. Intermediaries in the individual market, according to industry analysts, find it difficult to gather information and to obtain a suitable range of quotes for their clients (Laing & Buisson, 2004); if those with the appropriate qualifications and experience struggle to "shop around" in the market for PMI, finding the best-value deal is likely to be beyond the ability of most consumers.

The FSA had originally intended to include PMI under a separate category of "high-risk" product within general insurance, but the PMI industry opposed this and the FSA withdrew. A comment made by one member of the industry in March 2004 (echoing the Association of British Insurers' response to the first OFT report) captures something of the approach adopted by the industry during the consultation process: "it is clearly important", the speaker remarks, "to have some regulation, but too much is a bad thing". He goes on to say that "we have people complaining about lack of product innovation in the market, yet the regulator is telling companies what their brochures must look like. We shouldn't roundly endorse all regulation without appreciating that it does stifle innovation" (cited in Faherty, 2004).

This comment suggests that regulation of PMI sales could have some material impact on product design and product proliferation. The higher administrative burden on insurers and intermediaries under FSA rules could conceivably place a constraint on product differentiation if product differentiation were to become impracticable from the perspective of the sales person. However, it is too early to ascertain whether this is likely to occur. Moreover, given the marginal role played by intermediaries in the individual market for PMI, product differentiation would have to prove impracticable for insurers' own sales staff, and this is less likely to be the case, given that in-house sales staff do not have to present the products of competitors as valid alternatives.

Product development

The past few years have seen subscriber numbers in the individual market contract significantly, and those in the corporate market have begun to contract (see "Trends in level of demand over time" in Chapter 3). In the past, insurers have responded to market contraction by offering cheaper downgraded products in the individual market, and with highly competitive behaviour (including product underpricing) in the corporate market. It appears that these approaches have achieved all they are likely to achieve in terms of subscriber growth and retention, and, as a consequence, insurers are now looking for other ways in which to make their offerings more attractive to existing and potential customers.

Corporate market

Product development in the corporate market has centred on employee health management processes. This focus (promoting good health and identifying risk earlier on) could potentially lead to reductions in claims expenditure (or in claims expenditure growth), which could then be passed on to the employer in the form of a reduced premium. In addition, there is a possible benefit to be derived from employees being able to access a wider range of so-called "value-added services".

Norwich Union Healthcare, for example, now offers an online "Personal Health Management" tool as part of its range of corporate products: it enables employees to monitor their own health online and to access health advice. It also offers, to companies of 50 employees or more, an "Employee Assistance Programme", which gives employees access to a 24-hour helpline providing advice not only on health-related matters, but also on legal, financial, tax, personal, family and marital matters. The Employee Assistance Programme also enables employees to access counselling services. The "Platinum" version of the Programme, made available to companies with a staff of 300 or more, offers, in addition, special counselling for managers: this counselling can be of a personal nature or can relate to staff-motivation issues (*Cover*, 2004b). Another insurer, First Assist, offers a range of services that includes screening, occupational health services and access to physiotherapists, psychologists and rehabilitation services, as well as employee-training programmes and health-promotion programmes (*Cover*, 2004c). Such offers are now becoming standard across the market.

This health management approach can also form part of a wider, more integrated package of insurance-related benefits involving, for example, a health management presence in a company leading insurers to offer employers discounts on income-protection products designed to reimburse them for income loss owing to health-related employee absence (O'Doherty, 2004).

Individual market

The principal recent product developments in the individual market have been described above. They include, primarily, the development of cheaper products offering reduced cover, and the development of options such as restrictions on hospital choice and cost sharing. Product development has thus tended to focus on providing ways for the purchaser to obtain a lower premium as a result of reduced expenditure on claims.

Despite expression (within the industry) of the need to innovate on a more fundamental basis, most of the recent innovations have centred on making the standard product options more numerous or more sophisticated (including offering preventive-care options such as screening services). However, some recent products have been able to introduce new dimensions into product design, and insurers hope that these will help to reinvigorate the individual market for PMI. They include a product launched in 2005 by AXA PPP (and a similar one, launched previously by Freedom Healthnet), which combines PMI and critical illness cover in a single package, and the new product from Prudential which rewards health-improving activities with lowered premiums (*Cover*, 2004d; *Cover*, 2004e; *Cover*, 2004f). Meanwhile, Private Health Partnership has introduced a PMI product incorporating an investment component that functions to cover the excess payment (IFA Online, 2003) – in essence, a form of insurance-medical savings account combination of the type that appears to be gaining popularity in the United States health-insurance market (Robinson, 2002).

The direction product development is taking in the corporate market is much clearer than that in the individual market. In the corporate market, insurers are finding ways of better integrating the product into the everyday life of the firm by focusing on the preventive dimension of health care – something that is perhaps being facilitated by a broader workplace trend towards assuming greater responsibility for employee welfare generally.

In the individual market, however, the future of product design is less clear. The industry has recognized consumer concerns about value for money, and has also recognized the threat posed by the increasingly popular self-pay option (this development being facilitated by banks providing specialist health care loans and by hospitals offering different payment plans). Current trends in product development in the individual market appear, therefore, to be focusing on enabling customers to combine PMI with other private payment methods, and on enabling them to combine PMI with other insurance-related products such as critical illness insurance. These steps do not represent the radical advance that some commentators are suggesting is needed (and moreover, may serve to alienate less financially sophisticated clients).

Chapter 3

Demand for Private Medical Insurance

What drives demand?

In its insurance function, the NHS offers cover to all those "ordinarily resident" in the United Kingdom. Under the NHS, therefore, there is little uncertainty surrounding the possibility of financial loss resulting from the cost of health care per se. This means that other factors underpin demand for PMI. These factors are of two interrelated types.

The first relates to the price of PMI, and to perceptions about the quality of care provided by the NHS – in particular, perceptions about non-clinical dimensions of quality. The second relates to subscribers' personal characteristics. Studies have shown that PMI subscribers tend to share certain characteristics across the parameters of age, gender, area of residence, education, employment status, occupational status, political attitude, and income.

Research into determinants of demand for PMI makes use of data gathered from a range of surveys – principally the General Household Survey (Propper, 1989), the Family Expenditure Survey (Propper, Rees & Green, 2001), the British Social Attitudes Survey (Besley, Hall & Preston, 1999), the Family Resources Survey (Emmerson, Frayne & Goodman, 2001) and the British Household Panel Survey (BHPS) (Wallis, 2004; King & Mossialos, 2005). Earlier studies focused on demand for PMI in the individual market, but, as the corporate market has increased in importance, recent studies have covered both markets (Emmerson, Frayne & Goodman, 2001; Wallis, 2004; King & Mossialos, 2005).

Supply factors affecting demand

Satisfaction with the National Health Service

Consumer satisfaction with the NHS is difficult to measure, not least because there are conflicting views on how best to measure health care system performance. In studies of demand for PMI, the most common measure used is based on NHS waiting lists. In the mid-1990s, it was estimated that 20% of medical conditions generated up to 60% of PMI claims, by number, and that those conditions tended to be the ones associated with the longest NHS waiting lists (Natarajan, 1996). However, evidence about the overall effect of NHS waiting lists on demand for PMI is inconclusive.

Propper's work on demand for PMI, which looks at the individual market, has failed to find a direct association between NHS waiting lists and purchase of PMI. Her 1993 study (Propper, 1993) found no association between individuals' recent experience of waiting for NHS treatment and purchase of PMI, leading her to conclude that general perceptions concerning waiting lists may be more important than the actual experience of having had to wait.

Further work by Propper and colleagues (Propper, Rees & Green, 2001) again found little evidence of a positive effect of NHS waiting lists on PMI purchase. In fact, for most of the period studied (1978–1996), the estimated effect was negative – that is, waiting lists were associated with a fall in purchase of PMI. Spending on the NHS in previous years did appear to affect current demand for PMI, albeit with a time lag, but there was no clear relationship between the two. Overall, the study found that the availability of private-sector facilities locally, i.e. the number of private hospitals and the availability of part-time NHS consultants, was more strongly associated with demand for PMI than the total level of NHS resources or the lengths of waiting lists.

Using a different data set from Propper and colleagues – five years of the British Social Attitudes Survey rather than the Family Expenditure Survey – and controlling for corporate purchase, Besley and colleagues (Besley, Hall & Preston, 1999) were able to determine a positive correlation between NHS waiting lists and demand for PMI. Their study of data from the late 1980s and early 1990s showed that increases in long-term NHS waiting lists (12 months or more) were linked to purchase of PMI, and that if a long-term waiting list were to rise by one person per 1000, there would be a 2% increase in the probability of an individual with average characteristics purchasing PMI. The study found that the association between long-term waiting lists and PMI purchase was stronger in the individual market than in the corporate market, and that other NHS quality variables (such as waiting lists of less than 12 months or levels of public expenditure) were not significantly associated with demand for PMI.

Analyses of BHPS data find a statistically significant association between waiting times in the NHS and demand for PMI (King & Mossialos, 2005). King and Mossialos hypothesized that the effect of current waiting times was not specific to the wait in an individual's local health authority but was more likely to be a function of recent media reporting on waiting times appearing on a national basis. Like Propper, King and Mossialos suggested that the perception of waiting lists was more relevant than the actual experience of waiting, and that negative reports in the press would stimulate demand for PMI (with a time lag). However, their analysis found that the association between inpatient waiting times and demand for PMI was stronger, without any time lag being involved.

The King and Mossialos study also confirmed the finding by Propper and colleagues (Propper, Rees & Green, 2001) that the regional prevalence of surgeons with part-time NHS contracts is associated with purchase of PMI. An analysis of BHPS data (Wallis, 2004) found that although there did not appear to be any relationship between national waiting lists and purchase of PMI, there was a significant relationship between regional waiting lists and PMI purchase, indicating that individuals living in regions with high waiting lists are more likely to purchase PMI.

It should be noted that PMI coverage in the 1990s declined even though waiting lists continued to rise. Perhaps the most obvious explanation for this is that PMI premiums consistently rose above inflation, making affordability an issue for many existing and potential subscribers (Laing & Buisson, 2003). A report from 2000 found that while 40% of NHS users were worried about waiting for treatment in future and were concerned about declining service standards, the number of people purchasing PMI was only slightly higher in 2000 than in 1990 because many subscribers thought PMI cover was too expensive (BBC, 2000).

The AON Health Solutions survey of employers asked for employers' views on NHS waiting lists and service standards. The response showed that since 1998 there has been a considerable increase in the proportion of employers thinking that waiting lists will get shorter, and a small increase in the proportion thinking that NHS service standards will improve (see Table 3.1). Moreover, the survey found that between 1998 and 2001 "getting staff back to work quickly" had fallen as the main employer motive for purchasing PMI from a third to a quarter of respondents, although it was still the most important motive (see Table 3.4).

The price of private medical insurance

In the United States, demand for VHI has been shown to be price-inelastic (where an increase in price leads to a less-than-proportionate decrease in

Table 3.1 *Perceptions of NHS improvement under the Labour Government, 1998–2001, by percentage of employers (Source: AON Health Solutions, 2002)*

Measures	1998	1999–2000	2001
NHS waiting lists will improve	5.0	6.1	9.5
NHS waiting lists will remain the same	28.0	27.2	27.0
NHS waiting lists will worsen	33.0	34.3	28.4
Unable to answer	32.0	30.3	31.0
NHS service will improve	15.0	12.7	14.2
NHS service will remain the same	56.0	50.9	27.8
NHS service will worsen	24.0	31.8	25.6
Unable to answer	5.0	4.6	27.9

demand), being in the range of −0.03 to −0.54 (Manning & Marquis, 1996; Marquis & Long 1995). This finding may reflect the fact that in the United States VHI is largely employer-purchased, and is, moreover, subsidized by public funds (in the form of tax revenue forgone). The price-elasticity of demand for VHI in Spain has been shown to be similar, with one study of the period 1972–1989 finding it to be −0.44 (Murillo & Gonzalez, 1993).

In the United Kingdom, Emmerson and colleagues (Emmerson, Frayne & Goodman, 2001) found the price-elasticity of demand for PMI to be in the range −0.003 to −0.044, i.e. highly price-inelastic. The smaller effect of price on demand for PMI shown in this study may be related to the fact that PMI tends to be purchased by those in higher income groups and is otherwise provided to employees as a "benefit in kind". This hypothesis is supported by King and Mossialos (King & Mossialos, 2005) who, however, estimated a larger effect of price on demand for PMI among individuals aged 60 and over (at −0.50, nevertheless price-inelastic). Individuals in this group are substantially less likely to be covered by a company plan and are, therefore, as a cohort, likely to be more sensitive to price. The AON Health Solutions survey found that in 2001 73.2% of employers did not allow retirees to remain in the company plan, and that 56.1% of those who were allowed to retain their cover were retired senior staff (AON Health Solutions, 2002).

Tax subsidies

Although some European countries still use tax incentives to encourage the take-up of VHI (for example, Ireland and Portugal), in recent years there has been a clear trend towards abolishing, or reducing the use of, these incentives, as they have generally been found to be regressive, expensive and ineffective in terms of stimulating demand (Mossialos & Thomson, 2004). Governments use tax incentives if they wish to encourage the purchase of a product. Their use may be justifiable if the incentive is self-financing. The important question for decision-makers is, therefore, whether the savings to the NHS resulting from the take-up of PMI (as a direct result of the introduction of the tax incentive) outweigh the value of the expenditure or of the revenue forgone as a result of the subsidy.

From 1990 to July 1997, individuals aged 60 and over received basic-rate tax relief for the purchase of PMI. The removal of tax relief raised an estimated £135 million for the Exchequer in the 1999–2000 financial year. The removal of tax relief also led to a 29.9% increase in the price of premiums faced by the members of the affected group (Emmerson, Frayne & Goodman, 2001). Such an increase in the price of the premium might lead one to expect that there would have been substantial lapse rates among PMI customers and possibly a substantial increase in demand for services provided by the NHS. However, Emmerson and colleagues found that the decline in the proportion of the population aged 60 or over and holding PMI that could be directly attributed to the withdrawal of the tax subsidy amounted to only 0.7%, or to some 4000 individuals out of 555 000 (Emmerson, Frayne & Goodman, 2001). This finding confirms the low level of price-elasticity of demand for PMI, since a significant price rise led to only a small reduction in subscriber numbers. It also suggests that in the group comprising subscribers aged 60 or over, individuals are likely to belong to higher-income groups, where price-elasticity of demand for PMI is low.

These findings suggest that the policy of providing tax relief to individuals aged 60 or over was ineffective, as individuals receiving tax relief would have purchased PMI in any case. Moreover, although the change in the policy would have led to increased demand on the NHS, it is unlikely that this would have amounted to an annual value of £135 million.

Emmerson and colleagues also explored the issue of whether a tax subsidy for PMI in the United Kingdom could ever be self-financing: they found that an additional 1.8 million individuals would have to take up PMI for a subsidy to all adults equal to the basic rate of income tax to become self-financing. However, if the health care provided by the NHS also costs less than the health care provided by PMI (and Department of Health statistics suggest that NHS costs for treatment such as cataract surgery and hip replacements are approximately a third less than the same treatment on the private market), then an additional 3.1 million PMI subscribers would be needed to make the tax subsidy self-financing (Emmerson, Frayne & Goodman, 2001). In other words, in order for a subsidy to pay for itself in terms of sufficiently lowering the demand for the NHS, subscriber numbers would have to increase by an exceptionally large amount.

Subscriber characteristics

The personal characteristics most often associated with a subscriber to PMI relate to age, gender, income, educational level, employment and occupational status, area of residence and political attitude. Besley and colleagues (Besley, Hall & Preston, 1999) found that the typical subscriber to PMI is relatively well off, middle-aged and a supporter of the Conservative Party.

Age

Demand for PMI increases with age, but the association between age and PMI does not progress in a simple linear fashion, as demand peaks among individuals aged between 40 and 65 and is lowest for those aged over 70 and under 30 (Emmerson, Frayne & Goodman, 2001). Data from the BHPS suggest that demand for individual PMI is lowest among those aged 16–24 and highest among those aged 55–64, declining thereafter (Wallis, 2004; King & Mossialos, 2005). In 2001, only 2.7% of individuals in the 16–24 age group purchased PMI, compared with almost 8% in the 55–64 age group, 6.6% in the 65–74 age group, and 3.8% in the 75 and over age group (Wallis, 2004).

The non-linear pattern of age-related demand for PMI reflects the fact that younger age groups enjoy better health, while older age groups face supply-side constraints in purchasing PMI, including the higher cost of premiums for older people, the exclusion of pre-existing conditions and the tendency for employers to restrict retirees' access to corporate PMI. It may also reflect cohort effects. For example, Propper and colleagues (Propper, Rees & Green, 2001) analysed the Family Expenditure Survey data for the period 1978–1986 and found that younger generations are significantly more likely to purchase PMI than older ones, after controlling for personal characteristics and supply factors.

Data from the BHPS show that age and demand for PMI vary according to how PMI is held (King & Mossialos, 2005). In 2000, the average age of those with individual PMI was 50.7 years, 30.9 years for those with corporate PMI, 40.9 years for those with voluntary-group (company-organized but employee-financed – included in this report in the individual market) PMI, and 40.3 years for those covered by a family member.

Gender

Men are more likely to purchase PMI than women. According to an analysis of BHPS data from 1996 to 2002, men are almost three times more likely than women to purchase PMI in the individual market and almost twice as likely to be covered by corporate PMI (King & Mossialos, 2005), confirming similar

Table 3.2 *PMI coverage by age group for 1982–2001, as a percentage* (Source: *Laing & Buisson, 2003*)

Year	0–15	16–44	45–64	65+	All ages
1982	7	8	9	3	7
1987	9	9	11	4	9
1995	8	10	12	5	10
2001	N/A	14	15	6	12

N/A, not applicable.

findings made by all the earlier United Kingdom studies. However, these findings should be interpreted with some caution, as they relate to subscribers and not to family members to whom cover has been extended. Of the latter category, women account for 75.4% (King & Mossialos, 2005).

Income

Income has a clear and significant effect on demand for PMI, as demonstrated by all the United Kingdom studies, although its effect is found to decrease at higher income levels (Emmerson, Frayne & Goodman, 2001). Analysis of the BHPS data shows that individuals with higher incomes are more likely to have individual PMI – and more likely to have corporate PMI – than those with lower incomes (Wallis, 2004; King & Mossialos, 2005). Emmerson and colleagues (Emmerson, Frayne & Goodman, 2001) found that 41.2% of those in the richest decile have PMI compared to less than 3.7% of those in the poorest four deciles of the population, and that 50.7% of those in the top decile with PMI report that it was purchased by an employer compared to 25.5% in the bottom four deciles. This confirms an earlier study that showed that those with corporate PMI are typically wealthier than those without PMI and those purchasing individual PMI (Besley, Hall & Preston, 1999). Jobs offering higher levels of remuneration, therefore, seem more likely to offer other benefits, such as PMI. Studies also show that individuals with higher levels of savings are more likely to be covered by PMI, as are those who own their own homes (Besley, Hall & Preston, 1999; Emmerson, Frayne & Goodman, 2001).

Whether or not individuals live alone or with a partner or children has some effect on demand for PMI, which suggests that levels of disposable income may be more important than income alone in the decision to purchase PMI (King & Mossialos, 2005). For example, Besley and colleagues (Besley, Hall & Preston, 1999) found that PMI purchase is less likely among larger households. Similarly, Emmerson and colleagues (Emmerson, Frayne & Goodman, 2001) found that individuals living in households containing either adult children or unrelated individuals are 1.4 percentage points less likely to be covered by PMI than others. Other researchers (King & Mossialos, 2005) found that households with children are less likely to have individual PMI and less likely to have corporate PMI, but that individuals living with a spouse or partner are marginally more likely to have individual PMI and marginally less likely to have corporate PMI; however, these results were not statistically significant.

Educational level

Several studies have found that education is positively associated with PMI cover. Emmerson and colleagues (Emmerson, Frayne & Goodman, 2001) found that those with further education are more likely to have PMI than those who left education at the minimum school-leaving age. These findings are confirmed by BHPS data from 1996 to 2000, which show that those with post-secondary school qualifications are over six times more likely to have PMI than those without (King & Mossialos, 2005). However, extension of the analysis to incorporate BHPS data for 2001 and 2002 reveals that those with post-secondary school qualifications are only three times more likely to have PMI. The study by Besley and colleagues (Besley, Hall & Preston, 1999) concluded that social or cultural factors associated with newspaper readership appear to be important in determining demand for PMI, with readers of tabloid newspapers being less likely to purchase PMI relative to readers of broadsheet newspapers.

Employment and occupational status

Employment is an important determinant of demand for PMI. Employees are more likely to have PMI than either the self-employed or those out of work (Propper, 1989; Emmerson, Frayne & Goodman, 2001). BHPS data for 1996–2000 show that those in paid employment are more than twice as likely as those not in paid employment to have individual PMI (King & Mossialos, 2005). Contrary to expectation, Propper (Propper, 1989) found that being self-employed is negatively associated with purchase of PMI, but this result was not statistically significant. Besley and colleagues (Besley, Hall & Preston, 1999) also found that the self-employed are less likely to have PMI. However, analysis of BHPS data from 1996 to 2001 confirms the more intuitive hypothesis that the self-employed are more likely to purchase PMI (Wallis, 2004).

Occupational status also appears to be a key determinant of PMI coverage. Besley and colleagues (Besley, Hall & Preston, 1999) found statistically significant patterns in occupational data, with corporate PMI being particularly prevalent in financial services (21.9% of those with corporate PMI) and metals and mineral extraction (12.6%). The same study found that employment in the public sector is negatively associated with PMI purchase. AON Health Solutions reported that although the corporate market includes companies from all economic sectors, companies extending PMI cover to over 50% of their workforce are concentrated in the pharmaceutical, financial services, advertising/media, and communications sectors (AON Health Solutions, 2002).

Emmerson and colleagues (Emmerson, Frayne & Goodman, 2001) found that those in non-manual jobs are more likely to be covered by PMI, independently of their income, and that managers and technical staff are the most likely to be covered, followed by professionals and skilled non-manual workers. Members of the armed forces are the least likely to have PMI. The effect of occupational status on PMI prevalence is much more pronounced for corporate than individual PMI. For example, BHPS data for 1996–2000 show that professionals and managers are almost twice as likely to purchase individual PMI as unskilled workers or the unemployed, but more than nine times more likely to have corporate PMI (King & Mossialos, 2005). Corporate PMI is more common than individual PMI among professional, managerial and technical occupations, while individual PMI is more common among other occupations (Wallis, 2004). The greater prevalence of corporate PMI among men is consistent with the gender imbalance at higher occupational levels (King & Mossialos, 2005).

Area of residence

Data for 2002 from the Family Resources Survey show that individuals living in the south-east, London and the east are the most likely to have PMI, while those living in Scotland, Wales and the north-east are the least likely to have PMI (Laing & Buisson, 2003). PMI coverage ranges from 20% of the population in the south-east and 18% in London to 8% in Scotland, 8% in Wales and 6% in the north-east. King and Mossialos (King & Mossialos, 2005) found that those with individual PMI were less likely to live in London relative to all other regions in England, while those with corporate PMI were one and a half times more likely to live in London, but these results were not statistically significant.

Political attitudes

Several studies have shown that political attitudes influence the decision to purchase PMI. Besley and colleagues (Besley, Hall & Preston, 1999) found that individuals who support the Conservative Party are more likely to purchase PMI, and this is confirmed by analysis of BHPS data, which shows that those who vote Conservative are more than three times more likely to purchase individual PMI and more than two times more likely to have corporate PMI than those who vote for other political parties (Wallis, 2004; King & Mossialos, 2005). Other studies reveal that those who purchase PMI are more likely to be dissatisfied with the NHS (Calnan, Cant & Grabe, 1993) and less likely to be supportive of the equity goals of the NHS and increases in NHS spending (Burchardt, Hills & Propper, 1999).

Health status

The studies by Propper (Propper, 1989; Propper, 1993), which examined the impact of current health status on PMI coverage, did not find any clear relationship between health status – measured by variables such as GP visits and inpatient stays – and demand for PMI. Propper's 1989 study found that smoking was not significantly associated with PMI coverage, although an analysis of BHPS data found a negative association between smoking and having PMI (King & Mossialos, 2005).

Trends in level of demand over time

Since the early 1990s, around 11.5% of the United Kingdom population has had some form of PMI cover (this figure includes subscribers and their covered dependants). Table 3.3 shows subscribers, people covered and people covered as a percentage of the population for the individual market, the corporate market and the total market between 1990 and 2003. These figures are provided by industry analyst Laing & Buisson.

Industry analysts describe the market for PMI, as measured by level of demand in subscriber numbers, as having been relatively static for several years. Growth in the level of demand for the period 1991 to 2003 was –15% in the individual market, 30% in the corporate market, and 11.3% overall. For the recent cluster, 1999–2003, it was –10% in the individual market, 10% in the corporate market, and 3.11% for the market as a whole. In 2002 and 2003, the number of lapses (failure to renew) exceeded the number of new customers two years running for the first time, with a contraction in the overall subscriber base of 0.3% in 2002 and 1.02% in 2003.

It is clear from the figures provided by Laing & Buisson that the growth that has occurred in the level of demand for PMI has been driven by the corporate market – which, however, in 2003 contracted for the first time since 1994. Several factors are key to growth rates in the corporate market. These include the general economic climate – Datamonitor ventures that the contraction in the corporate market subscriber base in 2002 might be accounted for by the recent economic slowdown (Datamonitor, 2003) – the competitiveness of

Table 3.3 *Subscribers and people covered for 1990–2003 in the individual and corporate markets (Source: Laing & Buisson, 2004)*

Year	Subscriber Numbers (Millions)			Overall People Covered (Millions)			People Covered as Percentage of UK Population		
	Ind. market	*Corp. market*	*Total market*	*Ind. market*	*Corp. market*	*Total market*	*Ind. market*	*Corp. market*	*Total market*
1990	1.311	1.989	3.300	2.472	4.218	6.692	4.3	7.3	11.7
1991	1.366	1.934	3.300	2.570	4.077	6.651	4.4	7.1	11.6
1992	1.347	2.019	3.366	2.513	4.152	6.670	4.3	7.3	11.6
1993	1.327	2.065	3.392	2.440	3.909	6.351	4.1	6.8	10.9
1994	1.368	2.021	3.390	2.486	4.125	6.613	4.2	7.2	11.4
1995	1.408	2.022	3.430	2.558	4.115	6.673	4.3	7.1	11.4
1996	1.452	2.032	3.484	2.657	4.094	6.772	4.4	7.1	11.5
1997	1.378	2.108	3.486	2.392	4.277	6.679	4.1	7.4	11.6
1998	1.335	2.250	3.585	2.214	4.601	6.824	3.8	7.9	11.7
1999	1.285	2.275	3.560	2.121	4.415	6.536	3.6	7.5	11.2
2000	1.242	2.437	3.679	2.102	4.769	6.871	3.6	8.1	11.7
2001	1.216	2.506	3.722	2.049	4.621	6.671	3.5	7.9	11.3
2002	1.193	2.515	3.709	2.005	4.720	6.725	3.4	8.0	11.4
2003	1.157	2.514	3.671	1.956	4.679	6.635	3.3	7.9	11.2

PMI pricing, and employer attitudes to PMI. The reasons employers give for purchasing PMI, as reported in the AON Health Solutions survey, are shown in Table 3.4. A further factor affecting demand for PMI in the corporate market is the growing popularity of NIMES – a form of "self-insurance" that is exempt from insurance-premium tax. NIMES are a substitute for PMI, and further growth in this market will further reduce the potential for growth in the market for PMI.

Negative growth in the individual market has been significant: from a peak of 1.452 million subscribers in 1996, numbers had declined to 1.157 million by 2003. This contraction in the subscriber base can be related, in part, to the growth of the corporate market, with individuals newly covered by their employers giving up their individual cover (Datamonitor, 2003). It may also reflect other factors such as the removal of tax relief on PMI for those over 60 years old, the success of products such as health cash plans and self-pay, and large premium increases introduced in response to rising claims expenditure (Laing & Buisson, 2004; Datamonitor, 2003). Increased spending on PMI over the past few years, as measured by growth in insurers' premium income, appears, therefore, to reflect premium increases alone, rather than any significant growth in demand.

Laing & Buisson notes that, in the individual market, penetration among the higher-income groups reached a ceiling about five years ago, and attempts by

Table 3.4 *Principal motives for purchasing PMI, 1998–2002, by percentage of employers* (Source: *AON Health Solutions, 2002*)

Motive	1998	1999–2000	2001
To get staff back to work quickly	33.0	35.0	25.3
As a "perk" for employees	13.0	13.4	18.3
To keep the benefit package competitive	17.0	12.9	16.5
To ensure staff are well "cared for" during illness	20.0	22.7	17.0
To increase productivity	7.0	6.2	10.8
To reduce sickness-absence costs	10.0	9.8	10.1

insurers to expand into the lower-income groups by offering reduced-cover products at lower prices have largely failed to stimulate growth, instead serving only to help retain existing customers (Laing & Buisson, 2004).

Chapter 4

Supply of Private Medical Insurance: The Industry

Composition of the industry

The principal provider of data on the PMI industry is the analyst Laing & Buisson. In the two sections on the performance of the industry below, we take the Laing & Buisson data as our primary source. The first section describes the composition of the industry – the players, their market shares, and PMI distribution. The second focuses on the following three measures of industry performance: premium income, claims expenditure and gross margins. A third section ("Insurers and providers of medical services") looks at insurers' relationships with the other key component of the private health-care market, i.e. providers of medical services.

Providers of private medical insurance

In June 2004, there were 27 insurers operating in the market for PMI (Laing & Buisson, 2004). Only 19 of these were also providers of PMI. The remaining eight were not providers of PMI in their own right, but were providers of underwriting (or insurance) services to PMI carriers without an underwriting capacity of their own. Four of the insurer-providers were also providers of underwriting services to carriers. There were 15 carriers of PMI without an underwriting capacity of their own, and thus 42 players in all. The most important market players are all insurer-providers.

Historically, PMI has been provided largely by provident associations (whose profits are fed back into the company rather than to shareholders) based in the United Kingdom. The most important industry development of the 1990s was the entry into the market of commercial insurers, both United Kingdom-based and international. At the beginning of the decade, commercial insurers accounted for about 9% of the market; by the beginning of 1998, they accounted for 22%; at the end of the decade, the market share held by commercial insurers stood at about 50% (Laing & Buisson, 2004).

The two most significant commercial entries during the 1990s were Norwich Union Healthcare and Guardian Royal Exchange (Laing & Buisson, 2004). Norwich Union Healthcare entered in 1990, being the first large commercial company to do so. It achieved rapid growth in income (being largely responsible for overall industry-income growth at the beginning of that decade), but subsequent growth in the early 1990s was to come in terms of market share only and at the expense of that held by BUPA in particular (which saw its market share decrease from 44% in 1992 to 37% in 1997, before rising again more recently). The second significant entry was that of Guardian Royal Exchange, who entered the market in 1994 with the acquisition of Orion Healthcare. Guardian Royal Exchange went on to acquire PPP healthcare in 1998, before it was, in turn, itself acquired by the French insurer AXA (AXA's United Kingdom health business becoming AXA PPP healthcare).

It is sometimes claimed that the entry of commercial companies into the market during the 1990s led to a significant increase in competition within the industry. The full importance of commercial entry in terms of its impact on competitiveness within the industry is difficult to assess, however, as, barring the entry and rapid gain in market share of Norwich Union Healthcare, the distribution of market share at the top of the industry remained relatively stable across the 1990 watershed and has remained so since, with 78.5% of the market being concentrated in the top four companies in 1992 and 78% of the market being concentrated in the same four in 2003. However, it is likely that commercial entry did increase competitive pressures in the sense of forcing provident associations to mimic the market behaviour of the commercial companies (as far as we have been able to ascertain, there is currently little to distinguish the market behaviour of commercial companies and providents at the upper end of the market). But this change, in so far as it can be said to have taken place with any degree of certainty, may equally have come about in response to more general behavioural changes taking place within the wider business culture.

The early years of the new century saw two new patterns of entry emerge. First, 2002 saw health cash plan providers enter the market for the first time (for example HSA, Medicash and Health Shield). The second pattern to emerge in the new century was the entry of major insurers on an underwriting-only basis and, in an allied development, the entry of companies without a PMI underwriting capacity of their own. Insurers who have entered the market on this basis include AIG Europe, GE Frankona Re, Great Lakes Reinsurance (a subsidiary of Munich Re), United Life & Health Insurance Company (subsidiary of De Goudse, and underwriter to Freedom Healthnet) and Foresters, the only provident and the only United Kingdom-based company in this group (Laing & Buisson, 2003; Laing & Buisson, 2004).

PMI carriers who have entered the market on the basis of outsourced underwriting (and in some instances, outsourced claims administration too) include Berkeley Alexander, 21st Century Health Plans, HealthNow and – among entrants during 2003–2004 – Private Health Partnership, Patient Choice, Freedom Healthnet, Goodhealth, HSBC and Sainsbury's Bank (Laing & Buisson, 2003; Laing & Buisson, 2004).

The entry into the PMI market of insurers on an underwriting-only basis and of companies with outsourced underwriting and (in the case of HSBC and Sainsbury's Bank, for example) outsourced claims administration, together with entry via the joint venture, are the key features of a pattern that signals an increasing level of complexity and fluidity in the structure of the industry. It also signals continued confidence in the industry's prospects. Nevertheless, this new pattern must be set against a background of relatively low barriers to entry (and of costs related to exit) for companies willing to enter the market with outsourced underwriting and/or claims administration (although costs are higher for companies wishing to establish a secure presence in the corporate market).

Another significant recent entry into the market is FirstAssist, which acquired the health and accident business of Royal & SunAlliance in April 2003 in a management buyout financed by Barclays Bank and the Royal Bank of Scotland. The reason that this purchase was significant is not only that it signalled the market exit of a major provider of PMI, but that Royal & SunAlliance's health and accident business had been for sale since the beginning of the year without attracting the interest of the major established insurers – leading Laing & Buisson to comment that this instance of "failure to consolidate [within the industry] suggests that future consolidation in the medium term is unlikely" (Laing & Buisson, 2003).

The United Kingdom financial services provider Prudential recently entered the market in a joint venture with South African health insurer Discovery Health (with Discovery Health leading on product design and providing underwriting and management services). Part of Prudential's strategy is to offer discounted membership of health and fitness centres to its PMI customers (Laing & Buisson, 2004). Prudential has also established links with The Diagnostic Clinic, a provider of alternative health therapies (*Cover*, 2004f). Prudential's appearance is another instance of market entry on the basis of functions being shared across companies and across international borders.

The PMI industry has been marked by exits as much as by entries. Abbey National, the first major bank to enter the market (via a joint venture with Norwich Union Healthcare in 1997), transferred its share of the business to Norwich Union Healthcare and exited the market in 2001. Royal & SunAlliance, one of the leading insurers, exited in 2002 through a management buyout of its PMI business. Other companies to have exited the market include Private Patients and Bluesure in 2003, Allied Dunbar Healthcare, Healthcare-4-Life and Criterion in 2002, Lloyds TSB in 2001, and Ohra and Iron Trades in 2000 (Laing & Buisson, 2004).

Market shares

Table 4.1 shows the market shares, by premium income, held by the major insurers in the United Kingdom PMI market. It is clear that the distributions of market share among the top four, and among those immediately beneath the top four, have been relatively stable since the late 1990s. The figures presented are aggregated for both the individual and corporate markets.

The two largest insurers, BUPA and AXA PPP, continue to dominate the market, having more than 62% of market share between them in 2003. BUPA remained market leader in 2003 with 40% of market share – up significantly on 2002 and representing the third consecutive year of gain. AXA PPP remained in second place, with a decrease in market share masking an increase in profitability. AXA PPP's declining market share may be partly explained by the continued shedding of unprofitable business inherited from Guardian Royal Exchange (Laing & Buisson, 2004), and by the increasing attention it is giving to corporate-sector third-party administrator (TPA) business (see below) (Datamonitor, 2003) (income generated by TPA business will not show up as premium income in published company accounts). Norwich Union Healthcare remained in third place, with a stable 9% share of the market for the third year running.

On the basis of their survey of employers, AON Consulting report that, in the corporate market in 2003–2004, BUPA held a 45.5% market share, AXA PPP a 23.3% share, Norwich Union Healthcare a 6.6% share, and Standard Life Healthcare a 5.1% share (up from 4% in 2002–2003) (AON Consulting, 2004). The dominance of BUPA and AXA PPP in the United Kingdom PMI market, reinforced in part by their negotiating power with medical providers, means that publicity surrounding these two companies directly affects perceptions of the market as a whole (Datamonitor, 2003).

Table 4.1 *Market share, by company (percentage of overall premium income), for 1992–2003* (Source: *Laing & Buisson, 2004*)

Company name	1992	1997	2001	2002	2003
BUPA	44.0	37.0	37.0	38.5	40.0
AXA PPP Healthcare	28.0	29.0	25.0	23.5	22.5
Norwich Union Healthcare	3.5	7.0	9.0	9.0	9.0
Standard Life Healthcare	3.0	5.5	6.0	6.0	6.5
FirstAssist (formerly Royal and SunAlliance)	2.5	2.0	5.0	5.0	4.0
WPA	5.0	5.0	4.0	4.0	3.5
Cigna	3.0	2.5	3.0	3.0	3.0
Bristol Contributory Welfare Association (BCWA)	2.0	2.0	2.0	2.0	2.0
Total of above	91.0	90.0	91.0	91.0	90.5
All carriers	100.0	100.0	100.0	100.0	100.0

Third-party administrators and non-insured medical-expenses schemes

Although TPAs are neither insurers nor carriers of PMI, they are increasingly important industry players, being present in the corporate market as administrators of PMI schemes provided by insurers and as administrators of NIMES. According to Laing & Buisson, TPAs are often perceived to be more efficient in the administrative function than are PMI providers, and are able to be more responsive to company requirements (Laing & Buisson, 2004).

In recent years, NIMES have become an increasingly popular form of privately financed health-care cover in the corporate sector. NIMES are a form of self-insurance organized through a trust fund – set up for that sole purpose – into which the company makes payments and against which it makes claims to cover employee-related health-care costs (contributions into the fund being treated as taxable benefits). Companies may also take out stop-loss insurance with an insurance provider to manage the risk associated with unexpectedly high levels of claims expenditure.

The attractiveness of such schemes from employers' perspective rests on several factors. They are exempt from insurance premium tax and from FSA regulations dealing with capital requirements for solvency margins. They also avoid margins going to external companies, and they give employers a higher level of control over the design and operation of the scheme (Incomes Data Services, 2003). As AON Consulting advises the corporate readers of its survey, "self-insurance should be of interest to many organisations, with the increased flexibilities and tax efficiencies it can deliver" (AON Consulting, 2004).

In theory, NIMES can be administered by companies themselves, but in practice they are virtually always administered by a specialist TPA or by a PMI carrier operating as a TPA: AXA PPP, for instance, has recently been increasing its involvement in this type of service (Datamonitor, 2003). About 70% of NIMES are administered by PMI companies, with most of the remainder being administered by specialist TPAs (Laing & Buisson, 2004). For 2003–2004, AON Consulting found 5% of employers self-insuring, up from 4% in 2002–2003 (AON Consulting, 2004). Table 4.2 shows the significant growth in this area, with enrolee numbers, as a whole, growing more than 833% in 10 years.

As the example of AXA PPP shows, insurers have been keen to take advantage of the growing popularity of NIMES. Strong growth in NIMES, however, has coincided with poorer growth in the corporate market for PMI (where growth over the past 10 years, measured in subscriber numbers, has been under 22%). Adding NIMES figures to corporate market subscriber numbers would, of course, significantly increase the numbers of "insured" within the corporate sector, and across both markets it would mean that some 12.8% of the United Kingdom population is "insured", significantly above the 11.2% figure cited above.

Private medical insurance distribution

PMI can be sold directly by the insurer or through professional intermediaries. Intermediaries operate primarily in the corporate market, where there are currently over 100 firms active, and about 74% of all corporate market PMI sales are intermediated (Laing & Buisson, 2004). The main function of an intermediary is to select an insurer on the company's behalf; this is done on a commission basis or a fee basis. But the role of the intermediary commonly extends into other areas such as claims administration and product or benefits design. Intermediaries can also act as TPAs. Taking into account all forms of advice given by intermediaries, AON Consulting found that some 80.9% of employers made use of intermediary services in 2003–2004, and that this was up from 70.6% in 2002–2003 (AON Consulting, 2004). Laing & Buisson estimates that, for the market as a whole, 53% of all PMI sales (in terms of subscriber numbers) were conducted through an intermediary in 2003; of these, about 90% were in the corporate market (Laing & Buisson, 2004).

The percentage of individual market business (as measured in subscriber numbers) sold through intermediaries in 1999 was 13%. This rose to 23% in 2001, an increase accounted for by Laing & Buisson by intermediaries entering the market on an accommodation basis (dealing with existing clients rather than attempting to foster new business). The figure declined again to 15% in 2003, Laing & Buisson's explanation being the existence of better-developed online purchasing systems. Currently, most PMI carriers are able to offer quotations to potential customers via their web sites. These may be quotations

Table 4.2 *Non-insured medical expenses schemes: enrolees and people covered in 1992–2003* (Source: *Laing & Buisson, 2004*)

Year	Enrolees	People covered
1992	53 000	106 000
1993	74 000	152 000
1994	81 000	167 000
1995	113 000	242 000
1996	151 000	329 000
1997	152 000	333 000
1998	174 000	370 000
1999	303 000	554 000
2000	320 000	595 000
2001	387 000	704 000
2002	442 000	818 000
2003	472 000	880 000

for guidance purposes, based on simple risk factors such as sex and age, or more detailed quotations based on further information. There is also a range of consumer web sites that enable customers to compare products and prices across the industry and to order an application form. WPA is the only company cited by Laing & Buisson as offering online purchasing for fully underwritten PMI; other insurers offer online purchasing for PMI underwritten on a moratorium basis only.

There are currently about 3000 intermediaries – mainly general insurance brokers and independent financial advisers – selling small volumes of PMI in the individual market (Laing & Buisson, 2004). According to Laing & Buisson, intermediation has a smaller role in the individual market because of "the low commission rates compared with the corporate market, the difficulties in gathering product information, and time absorbed by obtaining numerous provider quotations for each individual". However, the introduction of higher commission rates and the production of intermediary information services and products (such as specialist data sources and web sites) (Laing & Buisson, 2004) may help to stimulate intermediary interest in the individual market in future.

In the individual market, about 85% of individual PMI policies sold in 2003 were directly by insurers on the back of press, television and radio advertising, direct mail, and sales people employed by insurers on a salary or commission basis (Laing & Buisson, 2004). Table 4.3 and Table 4.4 include all health and accident insurance business rather than just PMI, but they help to give a rough picture of how much is spent on advertising, and the relative importance

Table 4.3 *Advertising expenditure (health and accident combined) (£ thousands) in 2001–2002* (Source: *Datamonitor, 2003*)

Company name	2001	2002
BUPA	10 838	11 839
HSA	4 499	6 466
Norwich Union Healthcare	7 232	3 869
AXA PPP	3 432	2 119
Abbey National	N/A	284
Standard Life Healthcare	6	95
WPA	89	47
Royal & SunAlliance	14	12
BCWA	2	2
Total	26 111	24 734
Total market	N/A	52 431

N/A, not applicable.

Table 4.4 *Breakdown of advertising expenditure by channel (%) for 2002[a]* (Source: *Datamonitor, 2003*)

Company name	Press	Radio	Television	Direct Mail
BUPA	14.7	8.2	59.1	17.9
HSA	21.6	0.0	77.7	0.7
Norwich Union Healthcare	17.6	1.6	1.3	79.5
AXA PPP	34.3	0.0	11.2	35.2
Abbey National	0.0	0.0	0.0	100.0
Standard Life Healthcare	0.6	0.0	0.0	99.4
WPA	96.3	3.7	0.0	0.0
Royal & SunAlliance	100.0	0.0	0.0	0.0
BCWA	100.0	0.0	0.0	0.0
Total	18.6	4.2	49.8	25.8
Total market	15.3	3.3	30.8	49.3

[a] Not all rows total 100; we do not know why this is so. Because the header categories do not exhaust all advertising channels, it is possible that the missing advertising spend has occurred elsewhere (on billboard advertising, for example, which is widely used by AXA PPP).

different companies attach to different advertising channels. (HSA is included in these tables, but its advertising spend was primarily in the health cash plan market; Abbey National is included too, despite the fact that it no longer sells PMI.)

Industry performance

Premium income

Premium income, claims expenditure and gross margins are interrelated:

movements in one will tend to elicit responses in the others. Thus, an increase in expenditure on claims and a subsequent squeeze on margins will necessitate increased premium income if margins are to be maintained. Premium income can be raised by increasing the price of premiums – the low level of price-elasticity of demand for PMI, moreover, enabling insurers to lose a portion of the subscriber base and yet to increase overall premium income – or by increasing the number of subscribers. However, although an increase in subscriber numbers will raise premium income, it might not raise it sufficiently to offset allied increases in claims expenditure. Insurers look for ways to achieve a balance between these factors, which would allow them to maintain margins without sacrificing market sustainability through high subscriber loss.

Table 4.5 presents figures for the income generated by the industry in the form of premium income, broken down by individual and corporate markets; it also presents real growth rates (that is, growth rates adjusted for the RPI) for premium income for the two submarkets and for the market in its entirety.

The two principal factors determining premium-income growth are premium increases and growth in subscriber numbers. In 2003, there was very limited growth in premium income relative to the growth rates in 2000, 2001 and 2002. Growth for premium income across the market as a whole was 1.1% in 2003 (down from 7.3% in 2000, 6.4% in 2001 and 5.8% in 2002). Throughout the 1990s, premium-income growth was driven largely by price increases in the individual market against a backdrop of steady contraction in subscriber numbers. In 1998, premium income fell in the individual market – a fall attributed by Laing & Buisson partly to lapses in high-premium policies following the withdrawal of tax relief for the over-60s in 1997 (Laing & Buisson, 2004) – although Emmerson and colleagues (Emmerson, Frayne & Goodman, 2001) found the effect of the withdrawal of tax relief to be small.

The other notable outlier was the substantial growth in premium income in the corporate market in 2001, following higher-than-average premium rises for corporate PMI against a backdrop of only slowly rising subscriber numbers.

According to the figures presented in Table 3.3 (subscriber numbers) and Table 4.5, in 2001 the average premium faced by companies for each employee covered was £545 (premium income divided by number of subscribers) (note that this figure groups subscribers who do not have cover extended to their dependants along with those who do). AON Health Solutions, on the basis of their survey of 700 companies, published in 2002, reports that the average premium price per employee without cover being extended to dependants was between £251 and £300 in 2001 (AON Health Solutions, 2002). Incomes Data Services, on the basis of a similar survey conducted with 55 companies, estimated an average premium of £368 (for 2002) for employees whose cover

Table 4.5 *Premium income and premium-income growth, 1989–2003 (Source: Laing &*
Buisson, 2004)

Year	Individual premium income (£ millions)	Individual premium income growth (real) (%)	Corporate premium income (£ millions)	Corporate premium income growth (real) (%)	Total premium income (£ millions)	Total premium income growth (real) (%)
1989	452	N/A	498	N/A	950	7.6
1990	525	6.0	584	7.1	1 109	6.6
1991	609	9.4	674	9.2	1 283	9.3
1992	699	10.8	763	9.2	1 462	10.0
1993	764	7.5	785	1.2	1 549	4.2
1994	831	6.2	785	−2.3	1 616	1.9
1995	887	3.2	831	2.3	1 718	2.7
1996	970	6.7	903	6.1	1 873	6.4
1997	1 045	4.5	954	2.5	1 999	3.5
1998	1 040	−3.7	1 031	4.4	2 071	0.2
1999	1 118	5.8	1 106	5.6	2 224	5.7
2000	1 249	8.5	1 207	6.0	2 456	7.3
2001	1 294	1.7	1 367	11.2	2 661	6.4
2002	1 393	5.8	1 469	5.7	2 862	5.8
2003	1 438	0.4	1 540	1.9	2 978	1.1

N/A, not applicable.

was not extended to dependants. Incomes Data Services notes that extending cover to the employee's family can increase the price of the premium by a factor of up to 2.5 (Incomes Data Services, 2003). The £545 figure cited above is about half the figure for the individual market, where, again on the basis of the figures presented in Table 3.3 and Table 4.5, the average premium faced by an individual (again a figure grouping those who have not extended cover to dependants and those who have) is £1064.

Datamonitor explains this difference in price between the two markets by the higher level of competition in the corporate market and by the differing profiles of the populations covered by the two markets, with the individual market providing cover to a larger share of older individuals than the corporate market (with older individuals accounting for a large proportion of individual market claims) (Datamonitor, 2003).

The survey of companies carried out by AON Health Solutions found that, in 2001, some 47.1% of companies surveyed experienced premium increases of over 6% (AON Health Solutions, 2002). The Incomes Data Services survey reports that, in 2002, of 42 companies selected from the 55 surveyed, 11 (26.2%) saw their premiums increase by 16% or more, 10 (24%) by between 6% and 15%, and 8 (19%) by between 1% and 5%; meanwhile, 4 (9.5%) saw no change and 9 (21.4%) saw overall price reductions (Incomes Data Services, 2003). Although the Incomes Data Services figures show that there is no inevitability to premium rises, these reductions in price are unlikely to represent real reductions for the same product. The probability is that these figures show companies' willingness to opt for downgraded products (less insurance in the form of reduced benefits or higher cost sharing) in order to contain growth in, or to lower, their payments to insurers. In their most recent survey, AON Consulting reported that 42.6% of respondents experienced premium increases of 6% or more in 2003–2004 compared with 52.9% of respondents in 2002–2003 (AON Consulting, 2004), suggesting that insurers may now be concerned about the impact of premium increases on future corporate-market development.

Claims expenditure

Claims expenditure is perhaps the strongest driver of premium increases (and on the back of these, of premium income in a static or contracting market). Table 4.6 presents figures for claims expenditure broken down by individual and corporate markets; it also presents real growth rates (that is, growth rates adjusted for the RPI) for claims expenditure for the two submarkets and for the market in its entirety.

Growth rates for expenditure on claims were far higher in the early 1980s than during the 1990s and into the new century, with the 2003 rate of growth in claims expenditure being at its lowest for a decade. Several factors may have influenced this historical decline in rates of growth. Laing & Buisson mentions the introduction of coverage restrictions, treatment networks, care-management procedures, the termination of GP fundholding (with its incentives to refer patients to private providers where possible), the shift from inpatient care to day-case and outpatient care, and reduced coverage of high-risk subscribers following the withdrawal of tax relief for the over-60s in 1997 (Laing & Buisson, 2004).

Premium income has to be higher than claims expenditure if adequate margins are to be maintained in the absence of strong stock-market growth and high returns on the investment of premium income. In only six of the 15 years listed in Table 4.6 did growth in claims expenditure exceed growth in premium income (these were 1989 and 1990, 1994 and 1995, and 1998 and 1999). Immediately following these three two-year clusters, premium-income growth rates were comparatively high, suggesting that insurers were responding to high growth in claims expenditure (relative to income growth for the same years) and to the resulting squeeze on administrative spending and profit, with high rises in premiums.

Table 4.6 *Claims expenditure and claims-expenditure growth, 1989–2003* (Source: Laing & Buisson, 2004)

Year	Individual claims expenditure (£ millions)	Individual claims expenditure growth (real) (%)	Corporate claims expenditure (£ millions)	Corporate claims expenditure growth (real) (%)	Total claims expenditure (£ millions)	Total claims expenditure growth (real) (%)
1989	372	N/A	440	N/A	812	9.3
1990	440	8.0	542	12.5	982	10.5
1991	519	11.4	607	5.8	1 126	8.4
1992	553	2.8	647	2.7	1 200	2.8
1993	579	3.1	645	−1.9	1 224	0.4
1994	619	4.4	675	2.2	1 294	3.2
1995	661	3.1	727	4.1	1 388	3.5
1996	729	7.7	774	3.9	1 503	5.7
1997	772	2.8	814	1.9	1 586	2.4
1998	814	1.9	889	5.6	1 703	3.9
1999	882	6.7	952	5.4	1 834	6.0
2000	916	0.8	1 027	4.8	1 943	2.9
2001	972	4.2	1 097	4.9	2 069	4.6
2002	1 035[a]	4.7	1 170[a]	4.9	2 205[a]	4.4

N/A, not applicable.
[a] Estimated figure.

Industry gross margins

Gross margins are usually defined as the excess of premium income over claims expenditure, and are usually presented as a percentage of the former. In the insurance industry, premium income is invested in the stock market, and in a rising market returns can be high, enabling insurers to make a profit even when making losses on their insurance business (insurers may take advantage of high stock-market growth, for example by underpricing their products to try to gain market share or to increase overall subscriber numbers). Here, profit deriving from the investment of premium income has not been included in figures for gross margins. Table 4.7 presents gross margins for the industry as a whole (or, alternatively, average gross margins within the industry) for the years 1989–2003. It presents figures for the individual and corporate markets and for the total market.

Average gross margins across the industry rose marginally from 23.3% in 2002 to 23.6% in 2003, their highest level since the late 1970s (Laing & Buisson, 2004). The trough in margins in 1990 and 1991 can be explained by high claims figures in combination with a period of strong price competition (coinciding with the entry of Norwich Union Healthcare into the market), and these years were immediately followed by substantial rises in premium prices, bringing average margins to around 20%.

Table 4.7 *Gross margins (%), 1989–2003* (Source: *authors' calculations based on figures in Table 4.5 and Table 4.6 above*)

Year	Individual-market gross margins	Corporate-market gross margins	Total-market gross margins
1989	17.7	9.6	14.5
1990	16.2	7.2	11.5
1991	14.8	9.9	12.2
1992	20.9	15.2	17.9
1993	24.2	17.8	21.0
1994	25.5	14.0	20.0
1995	25.5	12.5	19.2
1996	24.8	14.3	17.5
1997	26.1	14.7	20.7
1998	21.7	13.8	17.8
1999	21.1	13.9	17.5
2000	26.7	14.9	20.9
2001	24.9	19.8	22.3
2002	25.7	20.4	23.3
2003	N/A	N/A	23.6

N/A, not applicable.

A second trough occurred in 1998/1999. In 1998, there was moderate growth in corporate premium income and negative growth in individual premium income. This led to margins for 1998 and 1999 being unacceptably low, at 17.8% and 17.5% respectively, and insurers instituted substantial premium increases during 1999 to compensate. BUPA implemented average rises of 14% and AXA PPP rises of between 10% and 49% (although AXA PPP's average was closer to 10%) (Laing & Buisson, 2004). Premium income growth increased substantially following these price rises, but, because of parallel growth in claims expenditure, margins were maintained at around 20%.

Laing & Buisson comments that the 1998/1999 trough "indicated that a proportion of PMI written was sold at too low a price, possibly in order to inject growth into the market and/or to secure market share. Industry sources also reported that there was a higher than usual lapse rate for the more expensive policies, particularly for healthier individuals who are less likely to claim" (Laing & Buisson, 2004). (It was around this time that downgraded products, precisely those likely to appeal to individuals with a lower probability of having to claim, were becoming increasingly available.)

Higher margins for individual PMI than for corporate PMI reflect the more intense price competition in the latter market and, despite higher acquisition and other administrative costs in the individual market, the ability of insurers to pass on price rises without significant reductions in subscriber numbers.

However, recent increases in corporate premiums have led to a narrowing of the gap in margins between the two markets. According to Laing & Buisson, most insurers reported a moderation of premium increases in 2003 (with average increases of between 5% and 10%) (Laing & Buisson, 2004).

The ratio of corporate-market to individual-market gross margins (taking 2001 as an example, 24.9:19.8, or 1.26) masks a significant difference between the two markets in terms of their respective contributions to overall margins. It will be apparent from Table 4.5 that while levels of premium income are broadly similar for both markets, the fact that the individual market covers less than half the number of people in the corporate market suggests that, on average, premiums are double the price in the former. At the same time, Table 4.6 shows that claims expenditure, too, is broadly similar within the two markets, suggesting that the cost of claims associated with members of the individual market is, on average, about double that associated with members of the corporate market.

However, a less cursory examination of the figures reveals that this apparent equivalence masks the fact that gross margins in the individual market are somewhat higher than those in the corporate market. Staying with 2001, the individual market covered 1.956 million people, and accounted for a premium income of £1294 million and a claims expenditure of £972 million – a premium income per person covered of (on average) £662 and a claims expenditure per person covered of £497. The aggregated gross margin per person covered in the individual market was £165. In the corporate market, 4.621 million people were covered in 2001, accounting for a premium income of £1367 million and a claims expenditure of £1097 million – a premium income per person covered of £296 and a claims expenditure per person covered of £237. The aggregated gross margins per individual covered in the corporate market was £59. At the level of the individual covered, therefore, the ratio of individual market margins to corporate market margins was 165:59, or 2.8, significantly higher than the aggregated 1.26 figure noted above.

Figure 4.1 plots gross margins for selected insurers since 1997, and includes the figure for United States insurers (aggregated) for purposes of comparison. Gross margins must be sufficiently high to enable the insurer to meet expenditure relating to underwriting and business operations and to allow profit to be made. Current margins appear to have enabled a level of profit sufficiently attractive to keep insurers in the market, although according to our interpretation of company annual reports a significant component of profit derives from returns on the investment of premium income.

Table 4.8 presents profit levels in absolute terms, and as a percentage of premium income, for six companies selected on the basis of the fact that their company

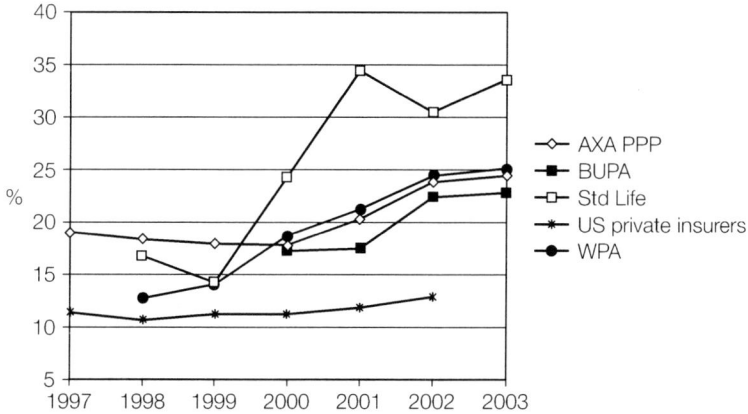

Figure 4.1 *Gross margins of selected United Kingdom insurers and United States insurers in 1997–2003 (Source: authors' calculations based on company annual reports and United States national health accounts data)*

annual reports present data for their PMI business that are relatively disaggregated from other business. It is evident that profit levels (including those calculated as a percentage of premium income) fluctuate significantly on a year-to-year basis.

Apart from generating profits, gross margins must be sufficient to cover insurer operating expenses or administrative costs. Because insurance company annual reports tend not to disaggregate their PMI business data completely from their other business data, there is no clear picture available of PMI-related administrative costs in the United Kingdom PMI industry. Table 4.9, which is based on the same insurers as in Table 4.8 (who do present relatively disaggregated data), provides figures for administrative costs in absolute terms and as a percentage of premium income. It will be apparent that, unlike in the case of profit levels (which vary from year to year), administrative costs, as a percentage of premium income, remain relatively stable.

Insurers and providers of medical services

As we noted above, financing by PMI flows principally to private hospitals and (to a lesser degree) to NHS private patient units and pay-beds. It also flows to other providers – providers of alternative therapies, for instance, or of home nursing services. This section focuses on flows of funds from insurers to care delivered in private hospitals.

Table 4.8 *After-tax profit levels for selected insurers in 2002–2003* (Source: *company annual reports and authors' calculations based on company annual reports*)

PMI carrier	Year	Profit (£ thousands)	Profit (% of premium income)
AXA PPP	2003	60 300	8.7
	2002	26 400	3.8
BCWA	2003	2 770	4.3
	2002	1 002	1.6
BUPA	2003	62 136	4.3
	2002	51 206	3.9
Standard Life Healthcare	2003	2 508	1.4
	2002	−2 404	−1.4
Provincial Hospital Services Association	2003	730	33.6
	2002	−830	−38.0
WPA	2003	12 520	12.1
	2002	4 464	4.1

Table 4.9 *Administrative costs for selected insurers in 2002–2003* (Source: *company annual reports and authors' calculations based on company annual reports*)

PMI carrier	Year	Administrative costs (£ thousands)	Administrative costs (% of premium income)
AXA PPP	2003	120 800	17.4
	2002	114 600	16.6
BCWA	2003	8 514	13.2
	2002	7 094	11.6
BUPA	2003	248 415	17.3
	2002	229 035	17.5
Standard Life Healthcare	2003	64 166	35.1
	2002	55 948	33.5
Provincial Hospital Services Association	2003	487	22.4
	2002	532	24.4
WPA	2003	18 894	18.3
	2002	16 715	15.2

There are five major private hospital groups in the United Kingdom. These are BMI Healthcare (with 44 hospitals), Nuffield Hospitals (with 41), BUPA Hospitals (with 34), Capio Healthcare (with 22) and HCA International (with six hospitals in London, among them the best known ones, such as The Portland, The Harley Street Clinic and The Wellington Hospital). There are also 93 private patient units located on the premises of NHS Trusts, and 40 smaller groups or independent private hospitals (Faherty, 2003).

Provider payment by insurers is comprised of two core elements: the facility charge and the specialist fee. In general, insurers reimburse the facility charge directly to the provider, whilst the specialist will bill the patient directly and the patient will then claim reimbursement from the insurer.

The facility charge

Private hospitals operate basic "rack rates", but actual charge levels are the outcome of confidential negotiations between insurers and providers, conducted on a bilateral basis. An investigation into the proposed merger of BUPA PMS [Private Medical Services] (now BUPA Hospitals) with the then-hospital group CHG [Community Hospitals Group] by the Competition Commission in 2000 reported that the actual charges set "reflect the bargaining strengths and abilities of the two sides, rather than the underlying structure of supply costs" (Competition Commission, 2000). Large insurers such as BUPA and AXA PPP therefore have an advantage over others when it comes to negotiating prices with providers, because of their size, experience and, in the case of BUPA in particular, their knowledge of private hospital operations and costs.

Speaking before the Competition Commission in 2000, BUPA said that it obtained, on average, discounts of 25–35% off provider "rack rates" for non-network business, and even higher discounts (the figure was not made available) for network business. The Competition Commission's own research showed that BUPA PMS charged BUPA PMI significantly less than it charged smaller insurers (with a difference of around 50% for knee operations), while BUPA PMS charges to AXA PPP for network business were, for three of the six procedures examined, 10% higher than its charges to BUPA PMI for non-network business. With respect to this variation, the Competition Commission commented that "it is far from obvious that the lower BUPA PMS charges to BUPA PMI [relative to AXA PPP] are fully justified on a volume basis or because of significant cost savings" (Competition Commission, 2000).

In its investigation of the proposed merger, the Competition Commission had sufficient concerns about competition problems within the market for private medical services (as that market related to PMI – from which, at the time of the investigation, it derived some 80% of its income) for it to recommend that the merger of BUPA PMS and CHG be prohibited. The Competition Commission's specific concern was that the proposed merger would lead to higher premium prices across the PMI market.

BUPA is the only company with a significant presence in both the private medical services and the PMI markets, and this was a source of concern to the Competition Commission, which felt that both BUPA PMS and BUPA PMI were gaining too much leverage from the relationship. Although BUPA denied that there was communication between the two companies of a type that could lead to unfair competitive advantage, the Competition Commission's investigation led it to lend little credence to the claim: "We are sure BUPA seeks in good faith to maintain Chinese walls", it noted, "but we do not believe that these arrangements can be relied upon: the external pressures are too great for their integrity to be sustained … We do not suggest that managers of the BUPA PMS and PMI businesses exchange price information: all that is necessary is for them not to adopt the sort of rigorous bargaining stances when dealing with each other that they would adopt when dealing with other providers" (Competition Commission, 2000).

Specialists

"The relationship between private practitioners and insurers", notes one commentator, "is a messy one, not least because of the lack of clarity surrounding fees" (Chapman, 2004). While insurers reimburse the facility charge directly, the subscriber is usually responsible for meeting the specialist fee and for then claiming reimbursement from the insurer. The level of fee that will be met for given procedures varies between insurers, who publish their fee schedules to their customers (apart from AXA PPP, who reimburses specialist fees at levels it defines as "usual and customary"). Any shortfall in the reimbursement of fees by the insurer has to be met by the subscriber (Federation of Independent Practitioner Organisations, 2003a).

In 1994, the Monopolies and Mergers Commission ruled that the guidelines for fees for named procedures produced for doctors by the British Medical Association "prevents, restricts or distorts competition in the supply of medical services" and that it was therefore illegal (Monopolies and Mergers Commission, 1994). In the same report, the Monopolies and Mergers Commission found that the benefits maxima employed by BUPA at the time – fee limits beyond which it would not automatically reimburse the subscriber – did not have a detrimental effect on the market for private medical services, and, moreover, that it constituted a "reasonable step" for the insurer to have taken (Monopolies and Mergers Commission, 1994). Insurers continue to voice frustration at fee levels, however (Baker, 2004), with one recent report finding specialist fees to be considerably higher than fees charged for comparable procedures by specialists in other countries (Bramley-Harker & Aslam, 2003).

There may be further factors at work within the provider payment mechanism. For example, in 1997 BUPA introduced its Consultants' Partnership Scheme (CPS) – a form of physician network, which required consultants to use one of the hospitals on the BUPA network even if the patient was a non-network patient, and which also required consultants to charge within the benefits maxima. In return, BUPA would pay the consultants a retrospective annual bonus amounting to 5% of the fees charged over the course of the previous year. In 2000, under investigation by the Competition Commission (see above) and subject to heavy criticism from the British Medical Association regarding the CPS, BUPA raised this bonus to 10% and the requirement that consultants on the CPS always use network hospitals was withdrawn (Competition Commission, 2000).

Sometimes consultants will have to be approved by the insurer before the insurer will commit to reimbursing their fees. It appears, however, that most consultants are on insurers' approved lists, and that this practice does not significantly restrict choice for subscribers.

In 2003, BUPA proposed the establishment of a list of preferred orthopaedic consultants – surgeons who would be "recognized" by BUPA to carry out hip- and knee-joint arthroplasty procedures. Inclusion on the list would be on the basis of a minimum number of procedures having been performed per year. The proposal also included the provision of a financial incentive to adhere to a BUPA-developed care plan. The profession's response to the BUPA proposals was negative, making nine key points, as listed below (Federation of Independent Practitioner Organisations, 2003b).

1 "BUPA should not dictate medical/surgical referral patterns. This is a fundamental principle." This proposal would undermine the referral role of the GP, who is best placed to choose the appropriate consultant.
2 "BUPA has no statutory role as a regulator of the profession". This response interprets BUPA as "setting themselves up as a quasi public body to license consultants to carry out specific procedures".
3 "The BUPA concept is not based on firm evidence and it is misleading to suggest that volumes of surgery done equate with quality in knee and hip surgery."
4 "BUPA has selectively modified the good practice guidelines for hip and knee surgery developed by the British Orthopaedic Association and the British Association of Surgery of the Knee". The profession states its support for appropriate clinical care plans, but indicates that these must not be "developed or modified by outside bodies who might be accused of having vested financial interests".
5 "The BUPA proposal includes an extra financial reward for consultants adhering to the specific insurance led plan and this may interfere with the consultant's role as the patient's advocate". The profession questions the ethics of this type of financial arrangement.

6 "The BUPA proposal implies a different standard of care for NHS and private patients". This is something that the profession does not accept.

7 "The BUPA proposal would exclude many perfectly competent consultants". For instance, experienced consultants (including female consultants and academic surgeons) who have reduced their workload could be excluded; it would also make entry into the market difficult for newly qualified consultants.

8 "The BUPA proposal will be a major disincentive to provide training opportunities for specialist registrars". This is because consultants needing to meet a certain target volume will be less inclined to offer training opportunities.

9 "The BUPA proposal will affect the introduction of new procedures".

The BUPA proposal combined two core elements of the managed-care approach developed in the United States: the preferred provider concept (already operative in the PMI market in relation to provider facilities), and the utilization review concept, whereby clinical provision is guided so as to achieve the delivery of cost-effective care. Managed care involves some restriction on clinical and professional freedom, and this partly explains the negative response of the profession.

However, a Market and Opinion Research International (MORI) poll found that some 38% of doctors currently providing services to PMI subscribers have some form of agreement with BUPA, or with BUPA and another insurer, with regard to fee levels (Federation of Independent Practitioner Organisations, 2004). BUPA continues to develop its relationships with providers in the direction of managed care, by seeking to establish episode pricing agreements (and moving beyond the facility/specialist fee separation), standard care pathways (including guidance on length of stay and the use of products and equipment), a reduction in fees in return for directed volume, a reward for increased productivity, and a focus on quality outcomes (Jones, 2004). Regarding the latter, since 1998, through BUPA Hospitals, BUPA has been operating an outcomes monitoring programme based on the "Short Form-36" questionnaire, which measures risk-adjusted health gain (physical and psychological) by having the patient answer questions before treatment and then some 12 weeks after treatment (Vallance-Owen et al., 2004; BUPA, 2004). The findings are intended to feed back into general care standards development processes and cost-effective provision within BUPA Hospitals, but strong evidence that the use of this type of survey, in circumstances of limited sample size and time frame, is an effective basis for quality improvement has yet to be presented.

Chapter 5
Conclusions

The state of the market for private medical insurance

Signals relating to the state of the market for PMI are conflicting. On the one hand, subscriber numbers are static – at best – or may even be declining. On the other hand, in 2003 gross margins were at their highest since the late 1970s, with growth in premium income exceeding growth in expenditure on claims by significant margins every year since 2000 (indeed, in 2003 there was barely any registered growth in expenditure on claims at all).

These gross margins reflect two factors. First, insurer successes in containing growth in claims expenditure – through wider use of cost sharing and other product options, the increased availability of downgraded products such as budget policies, prevention and promotion initiatives in the corporate market, success in the negotiation of provider charges, and caps on fee reimbursement to specialists. Second, they reflect the ability of insurers to institute substantial premium increases without adverse consequences in terms of subscriber loss, because of the low levels of price-elasticity of demand for PMI and because of the nature of the way in which insurers compete in the individual market, which makes it very difficult for consumers to "shop around" effectively for the best-value product. On the basis of gross margins, but in contrast with trends in subscriber numbers, the industry appears to be in good health – something confirmed by the continued level of interest in the market as reflected in the high level of market entry.

The principal threat to the health of the market is the decline in overall subscriber numbers (unless this begins to level off), and, in particular, the recent downturn in subscriber numbers in the corporate market, the sector upon which market growth as a whole has rested for many years now. Continued rapid growth in NIMES will also affect the potential for growth in the corporate market, and while these schemes are exempt from insurance premium tax they will continue to be attractive to employers. The one area where there is still potential for growth, according to industry sources, is the small-companies market (*Cover*, 2004b), for which there is likely to be a scramble among insurers in the coming years. However, it remains to be seen how successful insurers will be in encouraging the take-up of PMI in this sector, and whether small-company business will help them to maintain margins at current levels.

The presence of these threats may mean that the industry as a whole will suffer. Equally, it could mean, however, that the insurers with the largest market shares (BUPA, AXA PPP, Norwich Union Healthcare and Standard Life Healthcare) – who are also the principal providers of corporate PMI (AON Consulting, 2004) – will further consolidate their dominance of the market at the expense of smaller and newer insurers focusing on the individual market.

Despite trends in subscriber numbers, of particular note is the high proportion of the United Kingdom population with some form of privately insured access to health care. In 2003, some 11.2% of the population had PMI cover; adding figures for NIMES would bring the proportion of those with privately insured access to health care to some 12.8% of the population. In addition, some 8.1% of the population has a health cash plan (see the Appendix). (It is not known what proportion of these have a health cash plan in addition to PMI cover, but it will not be all of them, or even necessarily the majority.) The proportion of the population with private cover would no doubt be higher still if self-pay for privately delivered care were not becoming an increasingly attractive option as a result of higher incomes, hospital-offered payment schemes, specialist health care bank loans, and the perceived low value of PMI.

These figures show that a substantial proportion of the population (one that is usually ignored in the comparative literature) has some form of privately insured access to health care and, moreover, that insurers are currently not taking full advantage of this willingness to pay, either because they are not interested in doing so (it possibly being to insurers' advantage to forgo subscribers, especially those with a high claims probability, if this means that margins can be increased), or because they are unable to (although recent product innovations – apparently directed at the more financially sophisticated consumers, and possibly therefore at those at lower risk of incurring a loss – represent an attempt to do so).

Studies of demand for PMI show that subscribers continue to be concentrated among individuals of higher income, higher occupational status and in middle age. While there is some relationship between length of waiting lists or waiting times and demand for PMI, the connection is not as clear or as direct as it is sometimes assumed to be. It is therefore not possible at this time to say what effect the government's introduction of waiting-time maxima will have on demand for PMI in the future. It is equally difficult to predict the impact of government choice policies (including the option of publicly financed treatment in a private hospital) on demand for PMI. Moreover, reduced subscriptions to PMI may not necessarily reflect increased confidence in the NHS alone and may equally reflect the increasing availability of other forms of insured access to private health care or the increasing popularity of self-pay for elective treatment.

Issues for consideration

PMI is regularly presented as the archetypal form of supplementary VHI and yet it is little known. In this study, we have sought to provide a broad overview of the market, with two key purposes in mind. First, we aimed to provide an introduction to an often overlooked, under-researched and important component of the United Kingdom's health care financing mix. Second, we hoped to enable those with an interest in supplementary VHI to obtain a better understanding of how the United Kingdom market works. As we stated in the Preface, we have not sought to evaluate the market, nor have we sought to analyse its impact on the wider health care system. Data constraints – in particular, the absence of data on the internal operation of the market for PMI – have made any formal evaluation impossible. Nevertheless, some basic points likely to be of interest to decision-makers have been able to emerge, and, by way of concluding, we present these briefly here. These might be thought of as issues for consideration rather than as strong assertions.

(1) PMI operates alongside the public system of health care, to which subscribers to PMI retain full access. For this reason, PMI has been seen as an "extra" or as a luxury item, and has not been made subject to regulation (other than to ensure company solvency). Recently, the selling of PMI has come under statutory regulation (along with all other insurance sales), and this is likely to benefit consumers. However, in the absence of material (product and price) regulation (material regulation of supplementary VHI, moreover, now being prohibited under European Union legislation), the PMI market appears to behave as predicted by economic theory, namely, in a form that approximates monopolistic competition, with insurers competing through product differentiation (and proliferation) rather than simply on the basis of quality and price. This has been facilitated by the nature of pricing in this market, whereby personal characteristics affect the final price charged (since different insurers accord similar characteristics different values in the pricing equation). As a result, and taken together with the barrier to switching that is presented by the

receipt of treatment, the ability of the consumer to choose the most appropriate product may be severely constrained.

(2) Although PMI operates alongside the public system, it does not operate in isolation from it. Both privately financed and publicly financed health care draw on the same pool of medical specialists, and it is likely that developments or events on one side will affect the operation of the other. It is possible that the existence of PMI frees up resources in the public system, as patients opting to use their PMI are not using the public resources to which they have a right. However, it is also possible that because these patients are drawing on human resources that would otherwise be engaged in delivering publicly financed care, the existence of PMI may actually have adverse effects on the operation of the public system. This adverse effect might be manifested, for instance, in the form of waiting lists being longer than they would otherwise need to be among those who are unable or unwilling to pay to "go private". This is an important area that requires further research, but the evidence that is available (in particular, see Yates, 1995) suggests that adverse consequences are likely to outweigh any beneficial effects.

(3) Public systems, such as the NHS, which provide universal cover for a comprehensive range of benefits on the basis of need alone, tend to elicit public support for reasons that relate to equity (the efficiency arguments for such systems aside). They reflect a broad societal consensus around the existence of some form of (equal) social right to health care. In essence, the PMI market exists to "duplicate" certain of the services provided free of charge through the public system – albeit with enhanced non-clinical quality. It is arguable, on the basis of this essentially "duplicatory" function, therefore, that the existence of PMI does not undermine the equity objectives or basis of the wider health-care system. However, although in this study we have extracted non-clinical dimensions of quality from quality of care more generally, non-clinical quality and clinical quality cannot be entirely separated from each other. Clinical care always has a non-clinical quality dimension, and non-clinical quality might justifiably be considered a core component of clinical care (particularly, most obviously, as non-clinical quality can limit disease progression and aid recovery). If, then, some specified level of non-clinical quality is assumed to be fundamental to the care episode, the existence of a supplementary VHI market based on the United Kingdom model threatens the de facto emergence of what is usually referred to as a "two-tier health-care system" – thereby undermining the equity underpinnings of the wider health-care system as a whole. This process might be reinforced if patients were able to move seamlessly between the public and private systems in such a way as to allow them to benefit from the nature in

which the two systems interface – for instance, using PMI to "queue-jump" within the NHS.

(4) Arguments for providing public subsidies to subscribers to supplementary VHI are weak. Indeed, on the basis of the United Kingdom evidence, the only strong reason for providing such subsidies is to cater to a core-voter constituency. The argument for the provision of subsidies is that they would encourage the take-up of PMI and therefore relieve pressure on the public system, so that more resources are available to those who cannot pay for PMI. This argument is weak, both technically and ethically – technically, because subsidies go to those who would have purchased PMI in any case, and ethically, because these subsidies largely go to those in higher-income groups (funding access to better accommodation, better food, more-rapid treatment, and so on). Nevertheless, even without direct subsidies to purchasers, in a United Kingdom-type system of supplementary VHI, invisible public subsidies will inevitably remain in place. The existence of a public system to which right of access is universal means that (i) there is a back-up in place for when things go wrong in the private system, which means that those working in the private market are free to underinvest in expensive intensive-care services and technologies, to operate limited night-time staffing, and so on; (ii) insurers are free to focus on "profitable" services (routine elective surgery) and to ignore chronic care or other longer-term outpatient care; and (iii) insurers are free to risk-select their clients through the mechanisms of pricing, product design and exclusions. Do these issues matter? Perhaps not, but they might do. All three consequences may lead to distortions within the public system. In particular, in countries where public providers are being encouraged to operate "profitably", the self-selection of "profitable" patients and services into the private system on an organized basis might affect public system finances or service arrangements. Perhaps more significantly, there is the ever-present danger that a market in supplementary VHI will become more important than it was designed to be in terms of the provision of primary coverage. This is especially likely to be the case if its impact on the operation of the public system is especially adverse. Given the principle of actuarial fairness that governs supplementary VHI pricing, in conjunction with the market's freedom to select (services and risks), such a situation could lead to significant access problems further down the line.

Appendix – The Market for Health Cash Plans

Introduction

Health cash plans provide reimbursement for out-of-pocket payments for health care (or for other items relating to the use of health care). The benefit paid takes the form of a fixed percentage of the out-of-pocket charge faced by the subscriber, and there is an annual ceiling on the cash amount that can be paid in benefits for any defined area of health care (treatments and other items eligible for reimbursement are listed in the policy documents, as are items that are excluded from reimbursement).

For example, a benefit included in a health cash plan might be the reimbursement of 50% of all charges for dental care, up to an annual maximum of £100. If a subscriber visits a dentist and faces a charge of £80, he/she will submit a claim to the health cash plan provider (enclosing receipts) for the full amount. The provider will reimburse the subscriber 50% of the charge (£40). The subscriber can continue to make claims during that policy year until the £100 benefit maximum has been reached.

Health cash plan subscribers must usually be aged between 18 and 65, although providers may offer a separate pricing scheme to applicants aged over 65. Premiums are paid on a weekly, monthly or yearly basis, and range from about £1 to £15 per week (Datamonitor, 2003). Health cash plans generally provide cover for treatments that are not covered, or that are only partially covered, by the NHS – e.g. dental and ophthalmic care or complementary treatments. Many health cash plans also provide some form of cash benefit on the birth of a child or on the occasion of an overnight stay in hospital. A recent survey of health cash plans lists the following major categories of benefit: acupuncture, osteopathy, chiropractic, chiropody, homeopathy, physiotherapy, dental, optical, day-care admission, accident admission, surgical appliance and convalescent home (*Cover*, 2005).

Health cash plans may also provide cover for care that duplicates care provided by the NHS. Such cover might include, for instance, reimbursement towards the cost of a private specialist consultation. But claims of this type have been small in number historically and have largely been discouraged by the association representing providers of health cash plans (Gorsky & Mohan, 2004).

Health cash plans have their origin in the hospital contributory schemes of the second half of the nineteenth century. These schemes were popular among workers, both fulfilling a straightforward medical insurance function and providing a channel of funds to voluntary hospitals (which, nationally, received some 25% of their income from the contributory schemes) (Gorsky & Mohan, 2004).

With the arrival of the NHS and the tax funding of hospitals in 1948, about 200 schemes ceased operating. These were primarily smaller schemes affiliated with individual hospitals, but they also included some of the larger schemes whose members were committed to the tax-funded NHS and who feared that the continued existence of the schemes might undermine the NHS. At the same time, about 35 large city-wide schemes continued to operate. These tended to have considerable capital assets, strong roots in local workplace culture and a strong commitment to the voluntary sector (Gorsky & Mohan, 2004).

The survival and ongoing popularity of these schemes related to developments within the NHS. In the years following 1948, charges were introduced for NHS prescriptions, dental care and ophthalmic care, and the contributory schemes "reinvented" themselves (Laing & Buisson, 2004) to provide cover for non-acute care and care-related expenses, ceasing altogether to provide cover for acute care. Thus, although there were an estimated 10 million contributors to these schemes in the 1930s, in 1950 there were still some 3.5 million, despite the introduction of the NHS.

Market overview

Post-war demand for health cash plans peaked in the mid-1960s at about 4 million subscribers. This was followed by a gradual decline in subscriber numbers until a pick-up in 1989 and into the early 1990s, when the volume of demand stabilized at around the 3 million mark. According to Laing & Buisson, subscriber numbers remained static in 2003 at 2.892 million (with a further 1.904 million dependants being covered – in total, some 8.1% of the United Kingdom population), following small falls in 2000, 2001 and 2002 (Laing & Buisson, 2004).

As with PMI, health cash plans are offered in both the individual and corporate markets. Unlike the market for PMI, however, the great majority of health cash plans are held in the individual market (about 85% of policies). The share held by the corporate market, however, has been on the increase in recent years, from 8% in 1999, to 9% in 2000, 10% in 2001 and 15% in 2002. Most of this corporate business is concentrated among the major providers of health cash plans, e.g. Westfield and HSA. In 2003, there were an estimated 2.467 million individual subscribers and 421 000 corporate subscribers (Laing & Buisson, 2004).

Despite the origins of health cash plans in the lower-income socioeconomic groups, according to Datamonitor (2003) those people earning less than £15 499 per annum are among the least likely to hold a health cash plan, while those in the income bracket £40 000 to £49 999 are the most likely to have such a plan. By age, penetration is lowest in the 18–29-years group, and otherwise is fairly evenly spread (Datamonitor, 2003).

There are some 35 providers of health cash plans, 17 of whom also sell, or primarily sell, PMI. Twelve of these are non-profit companies, accounting for more than 90% of the market (the HSA Group alone accounting for almost half the market). In recent years, the market has seen some mergers and, despite static subscriber numbers, entry into the market by high street banks and supermarkets (Laing & Buisson, 2004).

There are various channels through which health cash plans can be sold, including direct sales, via brokers and independent financial advisers, and via employee benefit consultancies (Datamonitor, 2003). However, nearly all sales are made direct to the consumer (by in-house staff or sales representatives, through high street financial services retailers, by telephone or by mail and, increasingly, online); only 4.5% of sales are intermediated (Laing & Buisson, 2004).

Intermediated sales form a small proportion of total sales because, as health cash plans are low-cost products, commission rates for sales are low. However, with rising premiums and greater interest being shown by providers in penetrating the corporate market (where intermediated sales were up significantly from 2.5% in 2002 to 4.5% in 2003), interest from intermediaries may increase in future. Moreover, HSA, Norwich Union Healthcare and Legal and General have substantially increased the commission rates available to intermediaries, in an attempt to foster interest in this product (Laing & Buisson, 2004; *Cover*, 2005).

Variation in the advertising spend among providers is huge, with Birmingham Hospital Fund spending £46 in 2002 and HSA spending some £6.5 million

(Datamonitor, 2003). HSA's expenditure represented a 44% increase on the expenditure during 2001, much of this going on television advertising.

While subscriber numbers have been relatively static, with small declines in recent years, premium income has been on a continuous and significant upward slope (growing 33% since 1999). In 2003, income grew at its fastest rate since 1996, to 7.5%. Premium income in 2003 was £416.7 million (compared to £376.5 million in 2002). Broken down by sector, the individual market accounted for £353 million and the corporate market for £64 million (Laing & Buisson, 2004). This growth is attributable to premium increases, partly reflecting higher-value benefits (or product upgrading) and consumer willingness to meet price rises at this low spending base.

Since 1996, expenditure on benefits has been growing at a similar rate to premium income, with anomalies in 1999 and 2003 (in 1999, expenditure growth exceeded income growth by 3.2%, and in 2003, income growth exceeded benefits growth by 3.3%). Growth in benefits expenditure has been driven by rises in claims on the back of broadened coverage and higher payouts.

Of the £295.4 million benefits spend in 2003, £249 million was accounted for by the individual market and £46 million by the corporate market (Laing & Buisson, 2004). Table A.1 provides a breakdown of benefits expenditure, by category, for 2003.

Margins in 2003 were up significantly on margins for 2002, at 29.1% compared to 26.8% – their highest level since 1996 (see Table A.2). There is a greater degree of predictability in provider margins in the health cash plan market than in the market for PMI, as health cash plans provide limited cash benefits and providers are therefore better able to predict expenditure and to adjust premiums and benefits packages accordingly in order to maintain margins at desirable levels.

Laing & Buisson suggests that the industry may have made an aggregate operating profit (profit excluding income from the investment of premium income) of between £15 million and £17.5 million in 2003 out of these margins. This profit is up from about £10 million in 2002, and the bulk of it is held by HSA (Laing & Buisson, 2004). According to these figures, profit appears to have accounted for a little over 12% of gross margins in 2003. Therefore, a significant component of what are already high gross margins (29% compared to 23% in the PMI market) is accounted for by administrative expenditure. We cannot explain why this proportion should be so high, but we hypothesize that the nature of the claims process in the health cash plan market results in a higher administrative burden than that of the PMI market.

Table A.1 *Health cash plan benefits paid in 2003* (Source: *Laing & Buisson, 2004*)

	Proportion of total value of benefits paid (%)	Total category benefit paid (£ thousands)	Total number of claims (£ thousands)	Average benefit paid per claim (£)
Hospital inpatient	27.6	81 480	465	175
Optical	24.3	71 715	1 380	52
Dental	21.5	63 650	2 650	24
Physiotherapy	9.3	27 590	855	32
Specialist consultation	4.0	11 910	210	57
Maternity	3.0	8 930	39	228
Chiropody	2.5	7 465	650	12
Recuperation	2.3	6 855	80	86
Protection	1.9	5 650	3	1 750
Hospital day-surgery	1.4	4 205	145	29
Convalescence	0.8	2 405	5	531
Home help and illness	0.4	1 260	27	47
Hearing aids	0.2	585	7	81
Health screening	<0.1	125	2	70
Surgical appliances	<0.1	93	2	43
Prescription charges	<0.1	40	4	11
Others	0.5	1 480	28	54
Total	**100.0**	**295 450**	**6 550**	**45**

Table A.2 *Gross margins for health cash plan providers, 1995–2003* (Source: *authors' calculations based on figures provided in Laing & Buisson, 2004*)

Year	Industry gross margins (£ millions)	Industry gross margins (%)
1995	61.8	26.4
1996	78.8	29.3
1997	83.2	28.9
1998	90.1	28.9
1999	86.0	26.6
2000	92.8	26.9
2001	100.3	27.1
2002	101.0	26.8
2003	121.3	29.1

Glossary of Key Terms

Actuarial Fairness

A principle of justice according to which the price charged should correspond to the level of risk the insured person brings to the insurance pool.

Adverse Selection

A threat to the stability of insurance pools which derives from the presence of information asymmetry between the applicant and the insurer in the applicant's favour, such that it leads to the insured person paying less than the actuarially fair amount – and to others, as a consequence, paying more. This can lead to individuals who perceive themselves to be paying more than the actuarially fair amount withdrawing, and taking with them the subsidy their contribution was making to others. This, in turn, can lead to the pool coming to be comprised of individuals who cannot cover their expenditure on claims, and thus to the pool's collapse.

Co-insurance

The proportion of each claim that has to be met on an out-of-pocket basis by the insured individual, the insurer meeting the remainder of the claim. There may be an annual limit on out-of-pocket expenditure through co-insurance.

Excess

Also known as a deductible, this refers to the amount the insured individual has to pay towards the cost of any claim, the remainder being paid by the insurer. There may be an annual limit on out-of-pocket expenditure through the excess.

Experience Rating

Pricing on the basis of the previous year's claims experience, so that the premium reflects the level of claim experienced, adjusted for medical and general inflation and for the insurer's loading charge (covering administration costs and profit).

Hospital Network

A list of hospitals from which the insured individual is allowed to receive care under the policy he/she has purchased. Hospitals are included in a network if the insurer has managed to negotiate a discount on the prices the hospital charges.

Moral Hazard

A situation in which the fact of being insured leads to behaviour, on the part of the insured person, of a type that incurs costs but which, because it emerges after the fact, has not been factored into the calculation of the premium. The additional costs resulting from this behaviour have to be borne by the pool as a whole, thereby undoing the principle of actuarial fairness in pricing.

Private Medical Insurance

The term used in the United Kingdom to refer to supplementary voluntary health insurance. The term private health insurance is also used, although it is less common.

Product

The basic private medical insurance package, comprising a given set of benefits (or rights) and a price. Product options – for example, restrictions on how, or under what circumstances, private medical insurance can be used – can be added to the basic product, and the price will be adjusted to reflect this action.

Risk Rating

Part of the pricing process in an actuarially fair market, whereby applicants are assessed to determine the risk (the probability of incurring a loss) that they bring to the pool. Applicants are thus placed into different pricing brackets on the basis of standardized risk factors such as age and gender.

Underwriting

The process by which the insurer, on the basis of information provided by the applicant (and in some circumstances by the applicant's GP), determines the nature and amount of risk that it is willing to assume. For instance, if the applicant presents an especially high risk of requiring treatment for a given condition – because they have suffered from that condition in the recent past, or are suffering from it at the time of application – the insurer may choose not to extend coverage to this particular treatment.

Voluntary Health Insurance

Private health insurance the purchase of which is voluntary rather than mandated. Voluntary health insurance can be purchased by individuals, or by employers on their behalf. There are three types of voluntary health insurance. These are shown below.

Complementary provides cover for services not covered by the public system but that might reasonably have been covered under more favourable resource conditions, or provides cover for cost sharing within the public system.

Substitutive provides insured access to health care for individuals and groups not eligible for coverage by the public system (either because they have been excluded, or because they have exercised a right to opt out).

Supplementary provides insured access to health care administered and delivered outside the public system, without exempting the purchaser from having to contribute to the public system (to which right of access is maintained). The term "supplementary" refers not to the type of benefit covered but to the status of this system of insurance relative to the public system of coverage.

A wider glossary of insurance and insurance industry terms, as used in the United Kingdom, is available on the web site of the Association of British Insurers (www.abi.org.uk). The Insurance Information Institute (based in the United States) also provides a comprehensive glossary on their web site (www.iii.org).

References

AON Consulting. *Healthcare and risk benefits survey.* London, AON Consulting, 2004.

AON Health Solutions. *UK corporate health survey.* London, AON Health Solutions, 2002.

Armitage N. Paying as you go. *Cover,* Issue date: 1 June, 2004.

Association of British Insurers. *Are you buying private medical insurance?* London, Association of British Insurers, 2003.

BBC. Private medical insurance too expensive. BBC News, 5 October, 2000. (www.news.bbc.co.uk, accessed 25 August 2004).

Baker T. Contracting or employment of consultants. In: *FIPO report of meeting, 10 March 2004 at the Royal College of Obstetricians and Gynaecologists* (www.fipo.org, accessed 27 May 2004).

Besley T, Hall J, Preston I. The demand for private health insurance: do waiting lists matter? *Journal of Public Economics,* 1999, 72:155–181.

Bloor K, Maynard A, Freemantle N. Variation in activity rates of consultant surgeons and the influence of reward structures in the English NHS. *Journal of Health Services Research and Policy,* 2004, 9:76–84.

Bramley-Harker E, Aslam S. *Fees for medical specialists: how does the UK compare?* London, NERA Economic Consulting, 2003.

Bramley-Harker E, Lewis D. *Commissioning in the NHS: challenges and opportunities.* London, NERA Economic Consulting, 2005.

British Medical Association. Medical information and insurance: joint guidelines from the British Medical Association and the Association of British Insurers, 2002 (available at www.bma.org.uk, accessed 7 July 2004).

BUPA. BUPA calls for better measurement of healthcare outcomes. Press release, 27 April, 2004 (available at www.bupa.co.uk/about/html/pr/270404_outcome.html, accessed 25 May 2005).

Burchardt T, Hills J, Propper C. *Private welfare and public policy.* York, Joseph Rowntree Foundation, 1999.

Calnan M, Cant S, Grabe J. *Going private: why people pay for their health care.* Buckingham, Open University Press, 1993.

CancerBACUP. *Covering cancer: a review of private medical insurance policies for cancer care.* London, CancerBACUP, 2004.

CareHealth. Criticisms of private medical insurance by the Office of Fair Trading, 2004 (available at www.carehealth.co.uk, accessed 18 May 2004).

Chapman B. Private practice in the United Kingdom. *British Medical Journal,* 2004, 328:s15–s16.

Charitable Hospitals Federation. *Buying private medical insurance: information to help you and your family.* London, Charitable Hospitals Federation, not dated.

Chartered Insurance Institute. *Private medical insurance.* London, Chartered Insurance Institute, 2001.

Colombo F, Tapay N. *Private health insurance in OECD countries: the benefits and costs for individuals and health systems.* Paris, Organisation for Economic Co-operation and Development, 2004.

Comité Européen des Assurances. *Health insurance in Europe 1997.* Paris, Comité Européen des Assurances, 1997.

Competition Commission. *British United Provident Association Limited and Community Hospitals Group plc: a report on the proposed merger.* London, Competition Commission, 2000.

Cover. PPP adopts lifestyle underwriting for individual PMI. *Issue date:* 30 May 2003.

Cover (2004a). *Cover* survey. Individual PMI. *Cover Supplement,* Issue date: September, 2004.

Cover (2004b). *Cover* survey. Group PMI. *Cover Supplement,* Issue date: July, 2004.

Cover (2004c). FirstAssist launches new benefit range. Issue date: 1 August, 2004.

Cover (2004d). AXA outlines new PMI product. Issue date: 1 November, 2004.

Cover (2004e). Insurer Freedom Healthnet enters the PMI market. Issue date: 1 February, 2004.

Cover (2004f). Prudential sets sights on PMI market. Issue date: 1 September, 2004.

Cover. Cover survey. Cash plans. *Cover Supplement,* Issue date: April, 2005.

Datamonitor. *UK health insurance 2003.* London, Datamonitor, 2003.

Emmerson C, Frayne C, Goodman A. Should private medical insurance be subsidised? *Health Care UK* 2001, 49–65.

European Commission. Directive 2002/92/EC of the European Parliament and of the Council of 9 December 2002 on Insurance Mediation. *Official Journal of the European Communities,* L9/3 2003, (15 January).

Ewald F. Genetics, insurance and risk. In: McGleenan T, Wiesing U, Ewald F, eds. *Genetics and insurance.* Oxford, BIOS Scientific Publishers, 1999:17–34.

Faherty A. Choosing wisely. *Cover,* Issue date: 7 August, 2003.

Faherty A. New direction. *Cover,* Issue date: 1 March, 2004.

Federation of Independent Practitioner Organisations (2003a). *Medical fees in the private sector – an explanation for patients.* London, Federation of Independent Practitioner Organisations, 2003.

Federation of Independent Practitioner Organisations (2003b). *BUPA consultant orthopaedic preferred provider system for hip and knee joint surgery: a response by the medical profession.* London, Federation of Independent Practitioner Organisations, 2003.

Federation of Independent Practitioner Organisations. FIPO-commissioned MORI poll about independent practice. Federation of Independent Practitioner Organisations, 2004 (available at www.fipo.org/reports/mori_04_01.htm, accessed 27 May 2005).

Financial Services Authority. *Factsheet 2: Mortgage and general insurance regulation: what's changing.* London, Financial Services Authority, 2003.

Financial Services Authority. Insurance: conduct of business. In: *FSA Handbook.* London, Financial Services Authority, 2004a.

Financial Services Authority. *Insurance selling and administration: the FSA's final conduct of business rules.* London, Financial Services Authority, 2004b.

General Insurance Standards Council. *Practice Requirement E2 – private medical insurance.* London, General Insurance Standards Council, 2003.

Gorsky M, Mohan J. Hospital contributory schemes and health insurance in Britain, 1945–2000. Swindon, Economic and Social Research Council, 2004 (available at http://www.esrc.ac.uk/ESRCInfoCentre/index.aspx (use search facility for "Gorsky"), accessed 14 October 2005).

HM Treasury. Consumers and industry to benefit from changes to banking, mortgage and general insurance regime. Press release, 12 December. London, HM Treasury, 2001.

Higgins J. Incrementalism in UK policymaking on privatisation in health care. In: Maarse H, ed. *Privatisation in European health care: a comparative analysis in eight countries.* Amsterdam, Elsevier Gezondheidszorg, 2004:153–167.

IFA Online (2003). Hybrid insurance and investment product aims to cut cost of PMI. IFA Online, 2003 (available at ifaonline.co.uk, accessed 17 November 2004).

Incomes Data Services. *IDS Studies 745: private medical insurance.* London, Incomes Data Services, 2003.

Insurance Age. PPP launches new PDQ. Issue date: 1 June, 2003.

Jones R. What future private practice? [presentation] *FIPO Conference: UK Independent Medicine: Explosion or Implosion?, 10 November 2004* (available at www.fipo.org/docs/nov04/index.htm, accessed 27 May 2005).

Keen J, Light D, Mays N. *Public–private relations in health care.* London, King's Fund, 2001.

King D, Mossialos E. The determinants of private medical insurance prevalence in England, 1997–2000. *Health Services Research*, 2005, 40(1):195–212.

Klein R. *The new politics of the NHS.* Harlow, Prentice Hall, 2001.

Laing & Buisson. *Private medical insurance: UK market sector report 2003.* London, Laing & Buisson, 2003.

Laing & Buisson. *Health and care cover: UK market sector report 2004.* London, Laing & Buisson, 2004.

Lee P, Wallis G, Heasman D. Total UK health expenditure, 1997–2002. *Economic Trends*, 2004, 606:39–45.

Le Grand J. Further tales from the British National Health Service. *Health Affairs*, 2002, 21:116–128.

Lewis R, Gillam S. Back to the market: yet more reform of the National Health Service. *International Journal of Health Services*, 2003, 33:77–84.

Manning W, Marquis M. Health insurance: the trade-off between risk pooling and moral hazard. *Journal of Health Economics*, 1996, 15:609–639.

Marquis M, Long S. Worker demand for health insurance in the non-group market. *Journal of Health Economics*, 1995, 14:47–63.

Monopolies and Mergers Commission. *Private medical services: a report on agreements and practices relating to charges for the supply of private medical services by NHS consultants.* London, Monopolies and Mergers Commission, 1994.

Moss D. *When all else fails: government as the ultimate risk manager.* Cambridge, MA, Harvard University Press, 2002.

Mossialos E, Dixon A. Funding health care: an introduction. In: Mossialos E *et al.*, eds. *Funding health care: options for Europe.* Buckingham, Open University Press, 2002.

Mossialos E, Thomson S. *Voluntary health insurance in the European Union.* Copenhagen, World Health Organization Regional Office for Europe, 2004.

Murillo C, Gonzalez Y. El sector sanitario en España: situación actual y perspectivas de futuro. [The health sector in Spain: current situation and future perspectives]. *Hacienda Pública Española*, 1993, 119:41–58.

Natarajan K. *European health insurance markets: opportunity or false dawn?* London, FT Financial Publishing/Pearson Professional Limited, 1996.

O'Doherty S. Healthier attitude. *Cover*, Issue date: 1 February, 2004.

Office of Fair Trading. *Health insurance: a report by the Office of Fair Trading.* London, Office of Fair Trading, 1996.

Office for National Statistics. *Health: total UK health expenditure: latest estimates published as national statistics.* London, Office for National Statistics, 2004.

Office of Fair Trading. *Health insurance: a second report by the Office of Fair Trading.* London, Office of Fair Trading, 1998a.

Office of Fair Trading. Final warning to health insurers. Press release, 28 May. London: Office of Fair Trading, 1998b.

Office of Fair Trading. *Core terms products.* London, Office of Fair Trading, 1998c.

Office of Fair Trading. PMI and PMS markets are competitive says OFT but better information for policy holders is needed. Press release, 5 November. London, Office of Fair Trading, 1999.

Office of Fair Trading. Health insurers improve consumer information. Press release, 3 July. London, Office of Fair Trading, 2000.

Organisation for Economic Co-operation and Development. *Private health insurance in OECD countries: compilation of national reports.* Paris, Organisation for Economic Co-operation and Development, 2001.

Private Health Partnership. *Brief note on the main types of health insurance schemes currently available.* London, Private Health Partnership, 2004.

Propper C. An econometric analysis of the demand for private health insurance in England and Wales. *Applied Economics*, 1989, 21:777–792.

Propper C. Constrained choice sets in the UK: demand for private medical insurance. *Journal of Public Economics*, 1993, 51:287–307.

Propper C, Rees H, Green K. The demand for private medical insurance in the UK: a cohort analysis. *The Economic Journal*, 2001, 111:180–200.

Richards C, Dingwall R, Watson A. Should NHS patients be allowed to contribute extra money to their care? *BMJ*, 2001, 323:563–565.

Robb D, Brown P. *BUPA: 1968–1983: a continuing history*. London, BUPA, 1984.

Robinson J. Renewed emphasis on consumer cost sharing in health insurance benefit design [web exclusive]. *Health Affairs*, 2002, W139.

Saltman R. Melting public–private boundaries in European health systems. *European Journal of Public Health*, 2003, 13:24–29.

Seib C. Insurers are accused of leaving cancer sufferers in the lurch. *The Times*, 2004, 25 August.

Vallance-Owen A et al. Outcome monitoring to facilitate clinical governance: experience from a national programme in the independent sector. *Journal of Public Health*, 2004, 26:187–192.

Vallance-Owen A. Differentiating on quality [presentation]. *FIPO Conference: UK Independent Medicine: Explosion or Implosion?, 10 November 2004* (available at www.fipo.org/docs/nov04/index.htm, accessed 27 May 2005).

Walker S. Friend or foe? *Cover*, Issue date: 1 April, 2004.

Wallis G. The demand for private medical insurance. *Economic Trends*, 2004, 606:46–56.

Yates J. *Private eye, heart and hip*. Edinburgh, Churchill Livingstone, 1995.

Yates J. Memorandum by Professor John Yates: consultants' contracts, politicians' dilemma and patients' inequity. In: *House of Commons Select Committee on Health minutes of evidence: Session 1999–2000*. London, House of Commons, 2000.

Youngman I. *The health insurance opportunity: a worldwide study of private medical insurance markets*. Dublin, Lafferty Publications, 1994.

Index